Kind thoughts about Fr

CU00602229

*Tom is a true inspiration to al
someone with Alzheimer's and other forms of dementia. I admire
his ingenuity. He has managed to overcome grief, adversity
and a lost retirement by making caring for Margaret his 'fifth
profession'. Tom's book is a practical manual as well as being a
poignant insight into the everyday life of the unsung hero – the
lifelong carer.*

Richard Bagley,
Chairman, Thrive – a charity using gardening to transform lives
Director, The Roger Counter Foundation – a charity supporting
people living with lymphatic cancer.

*A moving and insightful account of one carer's very personal
journey which will resonate with many.*

*Tom details his caring experience from the start, writing about
the challenges faced, lessons learnt and people who have helped
to make a difference. This book will be of great support to family
carers at whatever stage of their caring journeys, and a useful
tool for all healthcare professionals that, in some way, encounter
dementia.*

Shemain Wahab,
Coordinator, Uniting Carers – an involvement network of
family carers of people with dementia,
Dementia UK – a charity intent on improving the quality of life
of *dementia* patients.

*Caring for a relative with dementia is very demanding, both
practically and emotionally. Tom Wearden's book is a thoughtful
and moving account of 15 years spent caring for his wife, which
brings the reader into his world. Anyone involved in dementia
care, either personally or professionally, will benefit from sharing
Tom's experiences.*

Linda Gabriel,
Chair, Bromley Mind – a charity providing dementia care and
mental health services in the London Boroughs of Bromley and
Lewisham.

Front Line Alzheimer's

Caring for Margaret at home

Tom Wearden

'The most powerful tools to help with the disease are
education, kindness and love...'

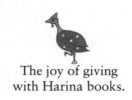

The joy of giving
with Harina books.

Front Line Alzheimers

Caring for Margaret at home

Text and illustrations copyright © Thomas Bertram Wearden.
tom.wearden@btinternet.com

First published by Harina & Co. (Publications) Ltd. 2013
a subsidiary company of Harina & Co. Ltd.
64 Baker Street, London W1U 7GB
www.harina-hanga.com

A CIP catalogue record of this book is available from the
British Library.

ISBN 978-0-9575386-1-0

Book layout, cover design, preparation and printing by:

York Publishing Services Ltd
64 Hallfield Road, Layerthorpe, York YO31 7ZQ
01904 431213
www.yps-publishing.co.uk

Contents

Acknowledgements

Since 1995 my learning curve has, at times, been very steep and I am indebted to the many healthcare professionals – carers, care managers, nurses, doctors, paramedics – from whom I have learned so much about Alzheimer's disease, and practical care procedures.

Amazingly, well over 350 people, including more than 300 visiting carers, have been involved in the network of support for Margaret that has built up.

I have mainly avoided mentioning professionals by name (there have been so many). However, I am especially grateful for a few important long term contributions.

Ruth and Ken Stannard, our neighbours across the road when we lived in Barton-on-Sea, became our very good friends. Ruth is a retired district nurse and Ken was a Police Inspector. They shared our day to day experiences as Margaret's condition worsened. Knowing that there was someone nearby to whom I could turn for practical support, help, advice or just a sympathetic understanding chat, was a lifeline for me. Ken (whose capabilities embrace wide ranging practical skills) undertook substantial work in the garden for several years, as well as dealing with a multitude of 'jobs' which, as a lifelong 'bodger', I had neither time nor ability to cope with. His help meant that I could concentrate my efforts on my main caring tasks.

Rhoda Curtis, our CPN (Community Psychiatric Nurse) in Barton, became our guide, guru, counsellor and friend from the time she first came to see us in 2001. Her regular visits, until she retired in 2009, were a lifeline for me. She was always able to provide informed professional information and advice about the hundreds of problems I encountered. Rhoda had a remarkable range of contacts within the NHS, Social Services and elsewhere; she was incredibly effective in calling for specialist back-up. She was one of those people whose influence and authority extended far beyond her status.

Sue Cooper was Margaret's chief carer in the Hampshire Social Services Home Care Team from 2003 to 2006. She worked closely with me to establish and develop practical care procedures. I learned a great deal about caring – and the caring community – from Sue. Since her retirement Sue has remained a personal friend.

Surangi Dissanayake, the senior carer looking after Margaret in the Bromley team was a senior nurse back in her home country, Sri Lanka, and brings great experience to her caring work. She has made a significant contribution to the development of caring procedures for Margaret and is an inspiring leader to the other carers. Surangi is another professional from whom I have learned a great deal about caring.

The carers

Our lovely, kind, considerate and eminently capable professional carers (Hampshire Social Services Homecare, Nov 2003 to May 2006, Willow Tree Homecare, May 2006 to August 2010 and HomeCare Bromley to the present day) are indispensable. Without their regular visits (two girls, three times each day) Margaret and I wouldn't be able to continue living together, sharing our lives in the way we do.

The family

I keep in touch by 'phone, almost every week, with Heather, Christopher and Mark. This is another lifeline, our family strengthened by their occasional visits.

The team

Finally, thank you to Cathi, Clare and Paula, of York Publishing Services, for their understanding, help and advice, to Ruth, Heather and Joy for reading and commenting on various parts of the text, and to my editors, Alicia and John Makin.

Tom Wearden
Bromley, Kent
August 2013

Introduction

In 1970 Margaret looked at me, sadly, after her mother's funeral. She said:

> 'Please, promise you won't send ME away to die like that, if I get Alzheimer's.'

We saw her mother, who'd had Alzheimer's for several years, a week before she died, in a ghastly mental hospital, where she'd been sent after her husband wasn't able to manage any longer at home. Her lovely curly hair had been cut very short. Many patients in the ward were partially dressed, shouting, pleading for help.

After seeing her mother's deterioration from being a wonderful, lively, bright-eyed caring lady, Margaret often spoke about her own fear of Alzheimer's. And she had nightmares, as well.

In 1998, 28 years later, my lovely wife showed the first signs. Early in 2001 she, too, was diagnosed with Alzheimer's.

The above is taken from my talk at the 2011 Dementia UK Congress. The text is reproduced in the last part of this book.

I'm Tom, it's 2013 and, when writing this book, I'm 83. I've cared for Margaret at home for 15 years. It's not the retirement with fun and travel that we'd both hoped for. But I've found some personal compensation.

There are hundreds of thousands of wives and husbands looking after their Alzheimer's stricken partners. I'm just one; we are all different. This is an account of my experiences.

Who? Why?

My book is mainly addressed to the many thousands of professionals – doctors, consultants, nurses, researchers, academics, social workers, even visiting carers – who interface in some way with Alzheimer's disease. Their work is often brilliant and inspired. Then they go home, hopefully feeling satisfied with a job well done. But I have encountered so many professionals who, despite their expertise and skills, have little or no proper understanding of the day-to-day life, anxieties, challenges and problems, faced by those who care at home for their Alzheimer's-stricken loved ones.

After my talk at the UK Dementia Congress 2011 I was amazed by the number of professionals, ranging from nurses to consultants and professors, who thanked me personally for illuminating parts of the overall Alzheimer's experience that they had never appreciated.

So this book is for all of us, too, my fellow carers, my colleagues around the world, hoping that we shall all benefit from better understanding by the professionals.

I was talking recently with an excellent visiting carer who asked if she could read my notes, made over many years, on which this book is based.

'What did you think?' I asked.

'Well, I'd never realised before that you grieve' she replied.

A few years previously I had asked a visiting carer if it might be possible to change the timing of the evening visit by half an hour. She turned on me.

"Why?"

"Because I would find it more convenient," I replied.

"We are here to look after your wife. Making things more convenient for you is not our job," she replied truculently. I gave up. Since this put-down, I never ask for any personal consideration from a carer or medical professional visiting Margaret.

And that's how it is, so often. To many visiting professionals, we devoted 24/7 home carers are wallpaper, without any right to life style, emotions or feelings. Their job is to look after their patients; ours is to quietly cope with whatever turns up, hopefully not making any fuss.

And then there are members of the lay public – friends, relatives, families who ask: 'What is Alzheimer's disease?' They hear and read radio, TV and newspaper reports that usually concentrate on the early year symptoms of memory loss accompanied by rather strange, even erratic behaviour. But I have found little public awareness of the way brain and bodily functions may be increasingly affected in later stages, to the point of total incapability. Is this because many Alzheimer's sufferers in the middle and late stages are incarcerated in care homes, where their deteriorating condition is hidden from the public and media?

This is not a textbook. I offer no medical knowledge or input except for the odd bits and pieces I have accumulated. But I hope that these notes about my experiences as 24/7 carer for Margaret help to explain what real life is like for many family carers who spend most of their time at the front line.

Understanding

Many text books and research papers with facts and theories about Alzheimer's have been published. I won't attempt a bibliography, but I must mention *The Daily Telegraph **Alzheimer's Disease*** by Dr William Molloy and Dr Paul Caldwell, first published in Canada, 1998, and first published in the UK by Robinson in 2002, ISBN 1-84119-474-3. A copy was given to me soon after Margaret was diagnosed in 2001. I bought several more for my family and others. It is excellent.

I am often asked about the terms 'Alzheimer's' and 'dementia'. I try to explain that Alzheimer's is the most common form of dementia. An understanding of Alzheimer's symptoms helps enormously in managing the lives of both the sufferer and the home carer.

Four essentials are:

Amensia – loss of memory.

Anomia – inability to find words.

Agnosia – loss of ability to identify objects and their uses.

Apraxia – inability to carry out purposeful movements.

If you are a home carer, try tossing one or two of these words into a conversation with a visiting professional. The result can be sensational.

In the early days, when Margaret still fed herself to some extent, all these symptoms were demonstrated when she was struggling to eat a bowl of breakfast cereal. She couldn't remember what she was trying to do (amnesia), say the name of the food (anomia), find the spoon and plate (agnosia) or fill the spoon and take it to her mouth (apraxia).

Before leaving definitions, I have used the conventional terms:

Home carers look after their patients 24/7 at home, without payment.

Visiting carers, often employed by specialist companies, arrive to perform specific tasks then go away.

There is some confusion because many organisations supplying visiting carers use the words Homecare or Home Care in their company names.

The beginning

So how did it start?

We were living very happily in Barton-on-Sea, New Milton, Hampshire, UK, where we had moved in 1982. After a marketing and management career in the electronics industry, I became a consultant and freelance writer in 1980 when I was 50. Our family had left home years ago and were more or less established. With this new independence Margaret and I, for the first time, could often travel and work together – she was a brilliant and meticulous proofreader for the reams of reports, articles and other written material I was producing. In 1997, aged 67, I slowly retired.

Then in 1998 came the first signs of Margaret's Alzheimer's disease. I love Margaret; how could I forget my promise to her in the 1970s? So I was determined to look after her at home for as long as possible. After all, Margaret had always looked after me – and our family. This was the start of pay-back time.

Now it is 2013. Margaret and I have been married for 58 years. She had always been a happy, feisty, loving person, laughing and bringing humour to those around her. But many years have passed since Margaret and I enjoyed a meaningful conversation. Even so, our love persists.

These are my experiences while sharing Margaret's Alzheimer's journey, as her 24/7 carer, for the last 15 years.

I started to record events and meetings – a habit from my business days – soon after her first symptoms appeared. By 2008 I was losing a lot of sleep because my mind kept going over and over the life we had happily shared and the many bad days as she deteriorated. So I started to bring everything together on my word processor, and the first part of this book emerged. Then, after we had moved to Bromley in 2010, to be nearer to our daughter Heather, I started to bring the text up to date and here it is in 2013.

Now

For many years Margaret has been doubly incontinent; she can no longer walk and has no purposeful movements. We have had no meaningful conversation since around 2002.

From late 2003, superb visiting carers have made sure that she is cleansed, showered and dressed. Amazingly, Margaret has been looked after by over 300 visiting carers in the last ten years.

The first were from the NFDC (New Forest District Council) Homecare Team; then in 2006 her care was contracted to Willow Tree Home Care Ltd. In 2010 we left the care teams that had looked after Margaret in Barton-on-Sea with many regrets. But, happily, here in Bromley she is very well cared for by the girls from HomeCare Bromley (formerly known as SureCare Bromley), the care provider appointed by Bromley Adult Services.

Margaret seems to be happy and still looks pretty. The doctors and district nursing team in Bromley are helpful and meticulous; everybody we have encountered has been welcoming.

She continues to enjoy her spoon-fed meals (her motto was always 'food comes first') and sips drinks (including sometimes a little wine at lunchtime) from a Doidy cup held to her lips. She sleeps for 22 or more hours each day. On a good day she will perhaps look at me and try to talk, but cannot find the words. (Doidy cups are shaped for invalids and children, available in many colours.)

But Margaret's beautiful smile persists. For her there is no past, no future, only the present, which changes as every second ticks by. Yet with her eyes she still manages to make those around her feel happy; and establishes a special communication with our children and with me.

When asked about her, there isn't much to say. I usually respond: *Inputs and outputs all working…*

or: *Things are as good as they could be, under the circumstances*. I find it difficult to say much more.

Caring is my fifth or even sixth profession. My career has included experience as an RNVR Officer, development engineer, sales engineer, company manager, business consultant and freelance writer; perhaps there are more that I have forgotten. At least I am accustomed to change.

In the early days of Margaret's disease I did everything; now my job is mainly concerned with housekeeping and making sure that we are well fed, that PC (personal care) is provided and implemented and that clean clothes and bedding are available. Every day is washday. My earlier 'hands-on' experience is invaluable now that the job has developed into a management role; I am able to take practical action, when needed, to make sure that everything happens as required.

And it certainly is a job. My first self imposed rule for staying more or less sane is to keep the 'the job' separate from the deep emotions that I experience.

My life since moving from Barton-on-Sea, Hampshire (where we lived for 28 years) to Bromley, Kent, is better. Our flat is new and manageable. I have all the time out ('respite' in socio-speak) that I can use; there is easy access to a wide range of shops, and we are only 15 minutes by train from London Victoria.

I see our daughter Heather (now 50) with Royston (our son-in-law) and her family regularly. Chris (Number 2 son, 53) in Bournemouth, and Mark (Number 1 son, 56) with his family, in Boston, Lincolnshire are accessible, without major expeditions. I am confident they would all rally round in a crisis.

I am always busy – this is essential! Apart from my interests in painting and music, I have revived some of my business consultancy work, which keeps my brain ticking over and stops me from moping around the place.

There is plenty to keep the adrenalin flowing.

Life in Barton-on-Sea, up to August 2010

Life in Barton-on-Sea, up to August 2010

Was this the beginning?

In 1995 Margaret and I celebrated our ruby wedding. We were married on 19th February 1955; our life together was – and still is – very happy. We have always enjoyed each other's company and tried to be together as much as possible. Our only disagreements were when Margaret complained that I was working too hard; I probably was. I was with various electronics and materials companies in sales, marketing and management roles, which involved travelling a lot with frequent visits abroad. In 1980 I became an independent consultant and also started to write articles for technical journals; these activities enabled us to live happily with more time together, as I was mainly working at home in Barton-on-Sea and Margaret could often come with me when I travelled.

Margaret had weighed nine or ten stone for most of our married life but late in 1994 she (unintentionally) started to lose weight and slimmed down to less than eight stone. This didn't especially worry me as she had had dramatic weight loss twice before, in 1959/60 and 1973/74. But in 1995 she started to have difficulty in swallowing and was often up at night regurgitating her food.

She was referred to the specialist who had cured her previous stomach ulcer problems (1985). After fibroscopy and barium meal tests no obvious cause was diagnosed. Metoclopramide was prescribed to help the muscles in the oesophagus work more effectively. Margaret has taken this drug ever since, before meals, firstly in pill form then later (when she started to refuse the pills) in liquid form that I mix with milk.

Margaret had always enjoyed her food, but lost interest as her appetite decreased. I started to take over the cooking and preparation of our meals, concentrating on a diet that could easily be digested. She gradually regained her weight and her appetite.

I don't know if this problem was an early symptom of her Alzheimer's disease.

Memories

In 1995-96 Margaret became increasingly vague; I was still working, and I recollect mentioning this problem to a client, when we were having lunch together, and to two or three people that I had met socially.

In the autumn of 1995 Margaret had an operation for varicose veins on both legs; looking after her for the next few weeks was somewhat stressful as she made little effort to co-operate. At the same time my eyesight was deteriorating.

In 1993 I had a cataract and lens replacement op on the right eye; now the same op was needed on the left eye. A date in December 1995 was fixed but in the hospital it was found that my blood pressure was too high and the op could not proceed. Pills were prescribed and my blood pressure was normal enough for the left eye operation to go ahead in March 1996. Margaret looked after me brilliantly during my recovery, with no obvious sign of memory loss.

It wasn't until 1997-98 that the first serious memory problems occurred. Margaret started to lose interest in selecting her clothes; she needed help in putting on her bra; she couldn't find her way out of the ladies toilet at Tesco's supermarket and had to ask for help. For many years Margaret had got out of the car and unlocked, then opened, the garage door when we arrived home after a drive. Suddenly she could no longer work out which key to use, or how to insert it in the lock.

In the course of my work I had generated a lot of written texts that Margaret meticulously checked, often suggesting simpler wording and looking out for repetition. In 1997 after I 'retired' I prepared a history of both our families (the Woods and the Weardens) and I also wrote a novel (everybody has at least one book in them). Margaret read and checked all this work. Her reading capability didn't diminish until later.

1998

Margaret was increasingly worried that she was going to get Alzheimer's. She very often talked and dreamed about how her mother died in hospital in 1970 a few years after being diagnosed with the disease. In January 1998 we saw our GP together and Margaret asked him whether she was developing Alzheimer's. He suggested that her loss of memory was just a natural progression at her age (she was then 67). She was reassured.

1999

I noticed that her interest in shopping and cooking started to diminish; I gradually took over so that by the end of 1999 I was firmly established as head cook and bottle (and clothes) washer. Margaret had always made sure the house was kept clean, asking me for help when needed, and she had done the washing. By 1999 she was uncertain what to do and we tackled the work together, aiming at a thorough house clean each month. She asked how she could help, but soon couldn't work out how to change pillowcases, or to fold washing.

By the end of 1999 I was dressing Margaret and helping her to wash, but she was coping with toilet visits on her own, with me standing by if needed.

2000

In July 2000 we had our last holiday. Christopher was living and working in Mallorca. He and his partner lived in a rented flat, and owned another, which we were able to use for a week. They looked after us brilliantly, taking us round to various places and entertaining us to superb meals. But Margaret was unhappy and soon wanted to go home. She didn't know where we were, or why. The adventurous spirit that had characterised our holidays for nearly 40 years, had disappeared. For the last few days in Mallorca we transferred to a hotel, which was a better arrangement; but I was concerned that Margaret would wander off while I was choosing meals for us at the buffet. We arrived back at Bournemouth airport late at night. It was obvious on the drive home that Margaret had no recollection of having been away.

Power of Attorney

I made enquiries about the procedure for setting up Power of Attorney (PoA) arrangements for the future. Our solicitors prepared the papers and obtained the signatures of the three eventual attorneys – Heather, our solicitor and me. The solicitor carefully explained the significance of the document to Margaret who then signed. The PoA was eventually registered in 2003, with medical support from our GP, when Margaret's condition was much worse.

Diagnosis

During 2000 there was continued deterioration; in November I spoke to our GP again. He referred Margaret to the Becton Centre in Barton-on-Sea. At that time, this was the Hampshire NHS Trust Locality Mental Health Team's Assessment Centre.

2001

In February 2001 we were visited by a doctor from the Becton Centre, who carried out the SMMSE Test (Standardised Mini Mental State Examination). I was still very vague about the nature of Alzheimer's Disease and the various types of dementia. The doctor told me she considered Margaret to be suffering from Alzheimer's. It was possible that progress could be slowed down by one of the drugs available, such as Aricept or the newer Reminyl; but the disease was already well advanced and it might be too late to consider this treatment. An appointment was made for a consultation with a Becton Centre consultant.

The Becton Centre sent us information about trials on these drugs, which suggested that there might be several side effects. Because of Margaret's previous stomach ulcer history I queried whether the treatment would be appropriate. The nurse at the Becton Centre said that Margaret must be prepared for a full medical examination; would I please make sure that this was understood? Margaret was adamant that she didn't want to see a doctor (she has always distrusted all doctors).

I spoke to the consultant by phone. Margaret was listening and saying loudly that she wasn't going to see him, and preferred to take her chances without treatment. Hearing Margaret in the background, he pointed out (not unreasonably) that there would be no point in proceeding with the appointment if Margaret did not come willingly. The appointment was cancelled.

Rhoda

Rhoda Curtis, the Community Psychiatric Nurse (CPN) based at the Becton Centre and responsible for outreach work, visited us soon afterwards. This introduction was the best possible outcome of the Becton Centre referral. Rhoda became our guide, guru, consultant and friend in the years from 2001 until her retirement in 2009. She visited Margaret every few weeks.

Rhoda contributed more than any other person or source to my personal steep learning curve. She is one of the most effective people that I have ever met, with an amazing repertoire of contacts that could be approached for solutions to problems which arise in looking after patients. Always kind and gentle, yet firm in her approach, Rhoda was very widely respected (perhaps feared!) by her fellow members of the caring community.

As Rhoda's visits came and went I had lists of questions for her (especially at the beginning) which she always answered with practical advice. The notes that I made before and during her visits have been extensively used in writing this account.

SCA Sitting Service

One of Rhoda's first actions was to put me in touch with the SCA (which then stood for Southampton Community

Association). Social Services have a duty to ensure that full-time carers get some free time, so we don't go completely potty. SCA activities included a sitting service, funded by Hampshire Social Services, which enabled me to have a few hours 'out' each week. This was how I encountered the socio-speak word 'respite'.

Jennifer

After an assessment visit by the SCA Manager in Lymington we were introduced to Jennifer who from 2001 to 2010 stayed with Margaret on days when I was out. At first Margaret would chat happily with her but over the years Jennifer saw and was saddened by her deterioration. Jennifer became a very sympathetic and understanding friend to me in a situation where finding someone to talk with is quite a problem.

A good read

In 2001 Ruth introduced me to a very readable book, *Alzheimer's Disease* by Dr William Molloy and Dr Paul Caldwell, which I mentioned earlier. This is the best book on Alzheimer's that I have read and I learned a great deal. It has helped me to anticipate and cope with the disease in its various stages as the years have gone by.

Increased disorientation

Margaret started to become increasingly disoriented during 2001. She was constantly looking for her mother. I had arranged to attend a 50-year reunion in September 2001, with several fellow ex-RNVR officers who joined the Navy with me for National Service in 1951. Heather (with Holly, her daughter) came to stay for the night.

Geoff Rigby, one of our group, had arranged the event. After a visit to HMS *Collingwood* at Fareham during the day we returned to our hotel in Portsmouth, where a celebration dinner had been booked. I phoned home to see if all was well; but Heather was very upset as Margaret had spent the day trying to escape. Eventually Heather and Holly had locked all the doors; clearly they weren't able to cope so I abandoned the dinner and came home.

Mirrors

Margaret started to find problems with mirrors. She would wave and talk to her own reflection (which I called 'Teragram' – Margaret in reverse). If she caught a glance of me through a mirror she would be frightened and say that there was another man in the room. This continued for several years and added to her overall confusion.

2002

Margaret had ceased to have much interest in clothes. I was taking her out to make purchases but soon found it much easier to buy from catalogues, in particular Ambrose Wilson, Daxon and Damart. I would select clothes from her wardrobe each day before washing and dressing her; every few days I would help her stand in the bath and wash her hair with the shower.

But on February 27 she collapsed into the bath with one leg underneath her. She couldn't make any effort to help me lift her up, so I called for an ambulance. The paramedic and the ambulance technician managed to lift her into their portable wheelchair, then helped her into bed. A visit to hospital was offered but I decided she would be better to stay at home, as there were no indications of any injury.

The ambulance crew then called out the duty doctor for a further check. No damage was found.

Going out to the shops was increasingly difficult. On more than one occasion, Margaret went to the ladies' toilet in Tesco's, then couldn't find her way out and had to ask for help in locating and opening the right door.

We went to the Pavilion Theatre, Bournemouth, to see 'Cococabana'. Margaret went first to the Ladies'. She didn't reappear for about 20 minutes; I was about to ask an attendant for help, but she emerged and said she had been waiting for me to collect her – inside the Ladies'.

2003

Early in 2003 Margaret started to be incontinent. Rhoda called in the incontinence nurse from the Practice, who visited us on February 05 and gave me advice on pads etc. She was a lovely person and came breezing in saying 'Hello, I'm the wee and poo nurse!' At first I bought these items but later the nurse arranged supply by the NHS, which has continued ever since.

Margaret soon became doubly incontinent. I was escorting her to the toilet, cleaning her, fitting replacement pads and generally making sure that she was able to continue with her habitual hygienic lifestyle. Margaret had mainly worn trousers but these became impractical so I started buying long Jersey skirts for her from various catalogues. Much to the later amusement of carers when they started coming, I used clothes pegs to hold Margaret's skirt over her shoulders when I was attending to her. In my own way I had made a contribution to care practice – several of the girls told me they had started to carry clothes pegs in their kit.

Margaret's mobility was already diminishing and I would set out a row of chairs from the lounge to the bathroom so she could sit down on the way, if needed.

Personality change

During 2002/2003 Margaret's personality changed. She had always been kind, lovely and understanding to me, but now became very hostile and argumentative. Nothing that I did was right. When I was looking after her in the bathroom, cleaning her after a toilet visit, she would say that there was no need as her mother and father would look after her. Conversation was becoming detached and very limited.

Toenails

One of the most difficult tasks was trimming and cleaning her toenails, because she tried to kick me away. I found a visiting chiropodist, who attended to this problem every few weeks. I held Margaret's legs still while she cut and trimmed. She was an ex-nurse with a good understanding of the situation.

Wandering

I had to watch Margaret carefully as she kept trying to look for her parents. One day I was doing some weeding in the garden and Margaret was watching me. She said she was going inside to wait for her lunch; I replied that I would be about ten minutes. When I went inside her coat was on the settee, but she was missing. I searched the house and looked round outside. I walked over to the cliff top. Ruth and Ken were out; I looked around their garden (where Margaret was convinced her mother lived).

Eventually I got into the car and found her in a side road asking people for directions to Westgate Drive where she had lived with her family, 250 miles away in Blackpool, until she left home to join the WRNS. She happily came home with me and we had lunch. After this I tried to be more diligent in ensuring that she couldn't go wandering.

Move downstairs

From 1982, when we bought our Barton-on-Sea house, we had slept upstairs in a bedroom with spectacular views across The Solent to The Needles. Worried about Margaret wandering in the night and possibly falling downstairs, early in 2003 I contrived a barrier at the top of the stairs. But it was clear that sleeping upstairs would soon be impossible. One day, much to the family's disgust as they thought I should have asked for help, I moved our double bed to the downstairs bedroom and took upstairs the twin beds we had for visitors.

I also transferred our chests of drawers. Matching wardrobes were already there. It was much easier to look after Margaret when we were sleeping and living downstairs, except that she occasionally strayed upstairs in the small hours, when I was asleep, still searching for her mother.

Shower room conversion

Washing Margaret was becoming a major problem and I decided to convert the downstairs bathroom into a shower room. Rhoda suggested that I should seek advice from Julia, the OT (Occupational Therapist) looking after part of the outreach work for the Becton Centre.

Julia had already been to see us several times; she had obtained a support with arms for use when Margaret was sitting on the toilet, and advised on many ways in which I could help to improve Margaret's lifestyle. Julia had pointed out the importance of tactile occupations, including the provision of old cards for Margaret to look at and generally fiddle with. She also suggested the purchase of special plates and cutlery to make it easier for her to feed herself.

Julia made a valuable contribution to defining our requirements; I obtained several quotations and eventually placed an order with Aquacare, the plumbing division of Bournemouth and West Hants Water Company (our local supplier). This company advised on the best makes of equipment to meet Julia's suggestions, orders were placed and they did a well-organised conversion of our downstairs bathroom, which took three days. We reverted to sleeping upstairs while this work was undertaken. Aquacare did a splendid, well organised and reasonably priced job.

I found out that the conversion would be VAT exempt and downloaded the relevant forms and regulations. I also found that the conversion of a second bathroom for invalid use, in a house with two bathrooms, qualified for a change in Council Tax band. This was agreed and we have enjoyed the benefit ever since, in Barton and later in Bromley. This reduction is not widely publicised – I only came across it by listening to the *Money Box* programme on the radio.

Desperate measures

Margaret was disturbed by the temporary move back upstairs. She was sick several times and became constipated – a condition that lasted for several days after we moved downstairs again. Over the previous few months she had vomited several times, mainly waking up in bed and covering everything within reach as well as having diarrhoea. On some occasions I had to change the bed linen and clean her up two or three times a night.

In October 2003, after ten days of constipation, she woke at about 2.00am in great pain. I walked her to the bathroom and sat her on the toilet; but, despite straining and bending, her bowels would not open. She was crying with pain. In some desperation I decided that this was a case for action with gloves and Vaseline. I was then able to help her with a manual evacuation. This did the trick.

Professionals would probably query this initiative (some have) but at 2.00am I couldn't hang around asking for advice or waiting for a nurse. I had previously spoken with our GP by phone; he prescribed Senokot which had just arrived, but Margaret hadn't yet taken a dose. I gave Margaret Senokot for several years after this event and the long term constipation didn't return.

Zoton

The GP prescribed Zoton (lansoprazole) tablets to prevent her regular night vomiting. I pointed out that Margaret by this time had great difficulty in swallowing tablets, so the Zoton came in a FasTab form which dissolves in the mouth. She has been taking these pills ever since and they have cured the vomiting problem which, I understand, was due to acidity.

Wheelchair

Rhoda suggested, in October 2003, that it would be sensible to order a wheelchair for Margaret so that it would be available when needed. Julia organised this and, when the chair arrived, she showed me how to install Margaret and manipulate the equipment.

It was first used early in 2004. We went for a walk (and ride) along Marine Drive, Barton-on-Sea. Margaret, by this time very disturbed, enquired whether I was trying to murder her.

Probus

In 1993 I had joined the Rhinefield Probus in Brockenhurst, a club for retired professionals and businessmen, which met for a talk followed by lunch on the third Wednesday of every month. Jennifer started by keeping Margaret company in 2001; I would leave a sandwich lunch for them as I was away for about five hours. But by mid-2003 Jennifer told me that, after about two hours, Margaret was becoming increasingly agitated by my absence. She was of course still mobile and Jennifer found her difficult to cope with. After reflection I decided that I should stop attending Probus meetings and agreed with Jennifer that her time would be split into shorter visits. This continued until we moved to Bromley.

Fast response

Rhoda visited us every few weeks and had often said that I should consider asking for help in looking after Margaret. Stubbornly I had maintained that I could cope on my own, but things were increasingly difficult as 2003 advanced. Eventually I realised that I would soon 'go under' and one day, when Margaret had been sitting on the toilet, then refused to stand still while I cleaned her up, washed her and sorted out her clothing, I phoned Rhoda. She was out but soon returned my call, at a time when Margaret was again loudly complaining while on the toilet.

I said to Rhoda: 'You were right. Can you organise some help please?' She could hear Margaret in the background trying to get up and asking who was on the phone, while still dirty and undressed.

Within two hours Rhoda had used her considerable influence and range of contacts to arrange for a carer from the Social Services Fast Response Team to come round and make an assessment. The first carer arrived on the following morning and together we helped Margaret to toilet and shower, get dressed and walk into the lounge for breakfast.

Risperidone

On the next day two carers came and this continued for two or three weeks until one day Rhoda phoned me. The Care Manager of the Fast Response Team had phoned her to say that Margaret had tried to strike one of the carers. The service would have to be withdrawn unless Margaret was immediately given tranquilliser treatment.

Rhoda sought my agreement then contacted one of our GPs. Ruth came to stay with Margaret while I went to collect the Risperidone that had been prescribed. The pharmacist explained that the dose, 0.25ml to be given 20 minutes before the carers arrived, had to be administered very carefully, using a pipette to accurately measure the quantity. A further dose was given 20 minutes before going to bed. The results were immediate and Margaret's hostility to everything (including me) reduced rapidly.

Homecare

After six weeks the Fast Response team passed Margaret's care over to Hampshire County Council Social Services Homecare Service. The Team Leader came and worked through the routine with me, then explained that initially they would only be able to provide one carer, who would work with me.

On the following morning Sue Cooper came into our lives. We soon established an excellent working relationship and she has remained a good and valued friend to Margaret and me ever since. Sue came on weekdays and Tania at weekends.

Several other Homecare girls joined the team looking after Margaret. We all got on well, with quite a few laughs – you can't do much else if you are working together toileting, showering, dressing and feeding an Alzheimer's patient.

Working with these down to earth and very capable girls every day, I learned a great deal about practical caring. I developed a deep admiration for the work of carers, a profession that I hadn't previously encountered.

2004

One or other of the Homecare girls was now coming every morning. Together we helped Margaret to get up and toileted, showered and dressed, then we walked her into the lounge where she was able to sit at the table for breakfast.

By early 2004 it was not possible for me to manoeuvre Margaret into the car and I abandoned all thoughts of taking her out for a drive again. Since then I have often felt lonely and sad when driving on my own, especially when doing something that Margaret always enjoyed, for example visiting a garden centre to buy flowers and plants.

Margaret often needed the toilet during the day. I helped her walk to the bathroom, first lining the route with chairs in case she suddenly decided to sit down. One of the girls brought us a Zimmer frame; Margaret wouldn't walk with this but I anchored her to it while I cleaned her, fitted a new pad and dressed her again as needed. We had also been provided with a toilet chair that fitted over the toilet. It had arms to prevent Margaret from falling sideways, and helped her to sit down and stand up.

TIA or fit?

On Sunday January 25, 2004 Margaret went into a sort of faint when standing up from the toilet; I sat her down again but couldn't bring her round, so I phoned for an ambulance which arrived within minutes. Margaret was still in a deep sleep; the ambulance people managed to lift her onto a stretcher then took her into the ambulance and gave her a whiff of oxygen. They advised me to let them take her to Lymington Hospital for a check over, to which I agreed.

Not knowing what to expect I gathered some night clothes together for her and drove to Lymington, stopping on the way to pick up a pack of sandwiches and a paper. Margaret was by this time lying on a bed in a side room from the emergency centre; I could hear her talking and as nothing seemed to be happening I went in to be with her. Eventually a nurse checked her with an ECG, and took her blood pressure, then a doctor arrived.

Basically they couldn't find anything wrong and decided to discharge her if she could walk reasonably well – which she could. A nurse helped me to get Margaret into the car and we came home at about 4.30pm. I made tea and Margaret behaved normally. We watched TV together until bedtime. She seemed to have no recollection of her visit to hospital.

This was the last time that Margaret went in the car.

Care home?

I was worried about the future. In early 2004 I contemplated arranging for Margaret to move into a care home. I discussed the options with Rhoda, who provided me with a list of establishments that might be suitable. But, on reflection, I decided that visiting Margaret in a home, trying to think of things to say, would be very sad for both of us. We were, and still are, closely attached; we continued to enjoy each other's company despite the adversities. And, after her mother's death, I had promised Margaret that I would do my best to look after her, avoiding despatch to a home, if (as she had feared) she developed Alzheimer's.

Move or stay?

Next I thought that perhaps the best thing to do would be to sell the house and move to Bromley, to be nearer to Heather and perhaps have some support from her. The house was put on the market and within six weeks an offer at the asking price came along. Heather looked round at possible flats and houses in Bromley. I arranged for a sitter, Jacqui, to look after Margaret while I went to spend a day with Heather.

She had made several appointments and I actually made an offer on a bungalow. However, on the train journey home I realised that this would be a bad move; and I found on my return that our purchaser in Barton had withdrawn his offer. Fate was clearly at work.

When I got back I found that Ruth, Sue and Jennifer had come to support Jacqui. It was clear to me that we should stay in Barton for the (then) foreseeable future. Care arrangements were already established; these might be difficult to replicate if we moved; and the general hassle could have been too much. I am often reminded of a well known inscription on a gravestone, much quoted by my father:

I was well, I wanted to be better – and here I am!

So I resolved to concentrate on organising life in our own home to be as comfortable and happy as possible for Margaret – and for me.

More TIAs or fits

Margaret's condition deteriorated in the first few months of 2004. On Thursday 29th January after her usual toileting, wash, and breakfast Margaret again wanted the toilet. The carer had gone by this time; I walked her through and she had a large BO (bowels open). I attended to her, then parked her on a shower chair (not the type with wheels that we have now). She started shaking – arms and legs – and her head lolled to one side. I brought in another chair and lifted her feet, which I had been told was the best procedure. She came round after about 20 minutes and was soon able to walk into the lounge where I sat her on a chair and she slept for the rest of the day.

I later found that this was either a TIA (Transient Ischemic Attack – a mild form of stroke) or a type of epileptic fit. Margaret has since had many more of these 'events'.

Negative risperidone proclamation

Towards the end of March 2004 it was decreed that Risperidone should not be given to patients with Alzheimer's, as it might increase the risk of a stroke. It was decided to withdraw the drug from Margaret over two weeks, starting with the evening dose on April 06 and cutting the morning dose on April 13.

Serious deterioration

On April 15 Sue and I couldn't wake Margaret. We tried to sit her up in bed but she wouldn't stay upright. We tried to help her stand but couldn't, so we left her in bed. Sue washed and changed her, then phoned the Team Leader of the Homecare girls to request an immediate increase in the frequency of visits.

I phoned the surgery. One of the GPs came; she could find no signs of a stroke – which I had feared – and Margaret's blood pressure was normal (133/83). Sue and Jane both came at lunchtime to wash and change her. She ate a small honey sandwich then slept again until teatime when she slowly ate a jam sandwich and had a drink of orange squash. Sue and Jane returned at 6.00pm, washed and changed Margaret again, then she slept through to eight the next morning.

When Sue came in the morning Margaret was very dirty and there were signs of blood; I phoned the doctor, who came in the afternoon. He said that there were several possible causes for the blood; investigation would be very upsetting to Margaret's quality of life. He saw lack of mobility as the major problem. Margaret stayed in bed. I bought a back rest to help in sitting her up, reducing the physical strain for the carers and myself. Ruth came over to see Margaret and helped me to fit the back rest.

Things continued like this until April 19. Margaret slept almost continuously, waking only for small amounts of food and drink, and for her PC. Two Homecare girls came to see to her, three times a day; this was the start of a new routine.

It has never been clear whether these events were due to withdrawal of Risperidone. I later (2011) found that this drug is still widely used as a tranquiliser, especially in care homes.

On April 19 Margaret seemed a lot brighter; we sat her on the edge of the bed and supported her while she stood for a few minutes, before returning her to bed. On the next day we were able to help her walk as far as the window and back. She continued to be very tired and spent most of the time in bed, but we persevered and walked her a little more each day. On April 24 she was still brighter. We were able to transfer her to her commode chair, wheel her to the lounge and then transfer her to the couch, where she stayed until the carers came again in the evening.

Over the next few weeks Margaret regained strength and we were able to resume her previous routine, but with the additional help from the carers.

Happier days

By June, 2004, it was clear that a lot of Margaret's previous hostility had disappeared; she was much calmer and generally serene. Rhoda suggested that this was because of the increased regular visits by the Homecare girls, which avoided the many arguments she had been having with me when I was coping on my own.

In May 2004 Rhoda and Julia suggested that we should have a hoist, so that it would be available if needed. The OT (Occupational Therapist) attached to Social Services came to see us for an assessment, then a manual hoist was delivered in July. The OT also arranged for the legs on our double bed to be extended, to make it easier for the carers to help Margaret out of bed.

Dental treatment

It was no longer possible for Margaret to visit a dentist; however I found that the NHS had a domiciliary dental service based (part time) in New Milton. We were visited on October 04 by Lucy, a very clever and understanding dentist, accompanied by her dental nurse. Margaret had bad decay is her lower teeth but any cleaning, filling and other steps could not be undertaken at home, so Lucy advised a strategy of prevention. I then made several changes to Margaret's diet. She also prescribed a special toothpaste, Duraphat, recommended for caries.

UTI

My attention was drawn by the carers to discolouration in Margaret's pads; a UTI (Urinary Tract Infection) was suspected. Sue and Rhoda were concerned, because a UTI is a special danger in Alzheimer's patients who may not have the resistance to prevent the infection spreading. I phoned the GP, quoting Rhoda who had considerable influence in medical circles. He prescribed an antibiotic. He was obviously concerned; one of the girls at the pharmacy said it was the first time she had seen him personally bring in a prescription. Ruth again came and sat with Margaret while I went to collect the medicine; Margaret was being treated within a few hours of the diagnosis and the problem cleared in a few days.

The carers had also reported traces of blood in Margaret's pads. Again I contacted the GP who said that he could think of six possible explanations. To find out the actual cause would mean an investigation in hospital which would be very disturbing to Margaret. The only time to worry would be if serious haemorrhaging occurred, in which case I should contact him immediately.

Golden Wedding

February 19 2005 was our Golden Wedding. Heather and Christopher had invited about 35 family and friends, and Heather organised a magnificent buffet lunch, including a beautiful cake that Chris had brought over from Mallorca. Chris made a super speech. Ken made sure that everybody had enough to drink. The room was like a floral hall! Happily the weather was fine, warm and sunny, even though it was February.

Margaret had four sisters; between them they had produced thirteen children including our three. Ten out of these thirteen cousins in the family came to the party – all adults now, of course, but I remembered them when they were children. Unfortunately Mark and his family were not able to travel down for the occasion. Margaret sat in a corner, in an easy chair, with two of the Homecare girls (Sue and Alison) who had volunteered to come and watch over her. Rita was a tower of strength helping to make everyone welcome in the reunited family gathering.

I think that Margaret took it in, even though it was all a bit overwhelming for her. She wasn't saying much by this time; the Anomia was obviously well advanced.

Eczema

Margaret had been suffering from eczema for two or three years. It had started when she was still able to visit the surgery, so it must have been 2001/2. The problem started on her right eyelid, then spread to her head and cheeks at both sides, then to her legs and feet. Various creams were prescribed. The most successful was Locoid Lipocream (hydrocortisone butyrate) which was suitable to be applied near to the eyes and at least kept the eczema under control; but the leg problem was not cured.

Margaret's niece, Mandy, came to the Golden Wedding and saw Margaret's legs. I explained the problem. Mandy has expert knowledge of eczema; I remember well how she suffered when a child. After a successful nursing career she was at that time sister in the Dermatology Unit at Harrogate Hospital. She described a treatment that she had used frequently: the affected area is completely covered with an emulsifying ointment, then another ointment, Elocon (mometasone furoate), is applied where there are patches of eczema. I asked the district nurse to come round and meet Mandy. She was then able to communicate the proposed treatment to our GP, who prescribed the two ointments. The eczema cleared within two weeks, after troubling Margaret for so long. I shall always be grateful to Mandy for her advice, which overcame a worrying problem.

Tom's health

In 1996 our GP prescribed Adalat because my blood pressure was high. In 2004 my left leg started to swell and furosemide was prescribed to reduce the fluid. However by February 2005 the daily swelling in my leg and left foot was quite painful by late afternoon.

The district nurse had a look when visiting Margaret and said I should be wearing compression hosiery. She made arrangements for me to be tested and Scholl's knee length socks were prescribed. The painful swelling was rapidly cured; I have worn these socks ever since.

Nights of delight

Margaret experienced BO problems in the late evening and early morning over many months. On one occasion I went to bed at around 11.30pm and found that she had had a severe attack of diarrhoea. On investigation, I discovered it was so bad that I had to cut her nightdress off, wash her, wrap a towel round and move her to a chair while I changed the bed, then back to the bed and put all the dirty clothes and bedding through the washing machine.

I felt that a large whisky was in order after this episode. And some people think I drink too much (comment from Heather: 'Others just join you').

There were many similar events. In the early evening – up to 9.00 pm – I could phone the Social Services Emergency Number. They were often able to find one of the Homecare carers to help me. Later, when Willow Tree took over (May 2006) there were several times when the girls came over to help in the early evening. But if the problem was in the late evening or early morning, I coped alone. Of course after Margaret became immobile, there was little I could do except change her on the bed, lie her on a towel, cover her and hope for the best until the girls came in the morning.

The job became easier when, later, a hospital bed was installed – except that the first time I tried to change her on my own at about 11.30 one night, I managed to get her knee stuck in the side bars. Learning on-the-job is all part of the caring game.

More TIAs or fits

During 2005 Margaret's condition continued to deteriorate. She had eight TIAs (or fits? which were they?) On June 23 Rhoda paid one of her regular visits; this time she brought her new Manager at the Becton Centre. They arrived to find that Margaret had flopped into the Glidalong commode chair and could not be roused. I had sent for an ambulance, which arrived shortly afterwards, manned by a paramedic who brought Margaret round with a whiff of oxygen then offered to take her to hospital for a check-up.

Instead I asked her to help me manoeuvre Margaret from the chair and into bed; she slept normally until the carers arrived at lunchtime to clean and change her, then slept all afternoon and was back to normal by evening. The new Becton Manager certainly encountered life at the front line for his introductory visit.

I alerted the doctor, who visited on July 04 after Margaret had been put to bed by the carers. He said it would be difficult to decide whether these events were TIAs or small epileptic fits – a condition often associated with Alzheimer's.

Shower chair

We were still walking Margaret to the toilet every morning, but sitting on the seat and standing up again was increasingly difficult. Julia, the OT from the Becton Centre came to offer advice. She arranged for a special wheel-along shower chair, with a horseshoe shaped seat, to be ordered by the Basingstoke based JES (Joint Equipment Service). Representatives from the manufacturer came to take measurements and agree on exactly what would suit best; a price was agreed with the JES. The chair was soon manufactured and delivered; it was in toilet service continuously until Margaret was no longer able to effectively use the WC (May 2007). However, use continued as a commode and wheel-in shower chair.

Margaret could be helped from the bed onto the new chair, wheeled over the toilet and then directly into the shower. After her shower the carers could help her to stand to be dried and then either wheeled or walked into the bedroom to be dressed and, finally, helped into the lounge for her breakfast. At first she would walk through (with help) and sit at the table, before being transferred to an easy chair to rest. As her mobility decreased the routine was modified until by May 2007 she could no longer walk.

The care taken by the JES in response to the needs identified and solution proposed by the OT illustrates the excellent help from the Hampshire JES that we experienced.

Reclining chair

Helping Margaret to stand up from an easy chair or the settee was increasingly difficult. I decided to purchase a reclining chair that would also tip up, so she would be more comfortable, and handling would be easier. One Friday, when Jennifer was sitting with Margaret, I visited the Red Cross Depot in Christchurch to look for a second hand chair.

By a remarkable coincidence, I spoke to one of the volunteer drivers who told me that he had recently been asked to dispose of such a chair by the relatives of a lady who had died. I followed him to his house in Christchurch, bought the chair (almost brand new) on the spot, and he delivered it later that day.

Di, the carer visiting Margaret at lunchtime, said that the sun had shone for me that day. I have never forgotten the phrase. Sometimes things just work out. The chair has proved to be superb and has greatly improved life for Margaret and all her carers (including me).

Bedding and hoisting

The Team Leader of the Social Services Home Care girls looking after Margaret came to see me in October 2005. She was concerned about the increasing difficulty in getting Margaret up from our double bed and, likewise, putting her to bed in the evening using slide sheets she had provided. I had made a point of personally trying out and experiencing all the caring procedures and routines, so that I could help when needed. I agreed that there was considerable strain in manipulating the slide sheets when working from the far side of the double bed.

She therefore proposed bringing in a hospital bed for Margaret, to which I happily agreed The hospital bed had to be ordered through the District Nurse Department of our surgery. A visit by the district nurse was arranged and, to explain the problems, I made a short film showing both the morning and evening procedures. The nurse was suitably convinced and immediately completed the documentation.

The electrically operated bed was delivered and installed by the JES on November 03. I had by this time ordered a single divan bed for myself; this was delivered on the same day by Bradbeers, New Milton, who also removed the surplus double bed.

I was very sad on the night of November 02 2005. Margaret and I had slept together for over 50 years. Margaret by this time had no idea what was happening, but I regarded the change in our sleeping arrangements as a significant milestone in her deterioration and an unhappy milestone in our married life.

A different hoist was delivered at the same time as the bed. This was used by for the first time on November 27 when Margaret had a TIA/fit, with copious BO, in the lounge while being moved to her reclining chair. The supposedly plain carpets in our house were generously decorated with random patterns resulting from this and similar events. It's all part of the caring scenario.

The manual hoist was not used regularly until later in 2006, as the hospital bed made it much easier to manoeuvre Margaret manually in the mornings and evenings.

Alzheimer's Society

Soon after Margaret was officially diagnosed in 2001 I made enquiries about the Alzheimer's Society and we were visited by a charming lady who lived in Lymington and was, at that time, the volunteer local representative. She explained the workings of the Society and subsequently I filled in the forms and joined. The regular publications were interesting, and I realised that I was not alone.

In 2005 I invited the new outreach worker from the New Milton Office to come and meet us. After discussion she suggested that I might like to consider joining the Alzheimer's Society QRD (Quality Research in Dementia) Network. I applied and was accepted.

The Alzheimer's Society provides substantial funds for relevant research projects, mainly in UK universities and hospitals. Many research proposals and applications for grants are received. After initial consideration, the most likely of these are sent for comment to members of the QRD network, all of whom have practical experience of Alzheimer's, as carers, relatives, healthcare professional and in other ways. I received a bundle of 5-10 proposals each month, with a score sheet 1-10 and an opportunity to make comments, anonymously.

The value or otherwise of many proposals is clear; but others are highly technical and I offered a judgment about whether the end result is likely to help Alzheimer's sufferers within a reasonable timescale. I also offered my view as to whether the proposer was likely to achieve something positive – or was the grant intended to prolong his/her life wandering up and down the dusty corridors of academia?

Sometimes the proposals seemed to have no logical foundation; on other occasions, if the project were to be successful, the cost of using the result on real-life patients would be prohibitive (for example the multiple use of expensive scanners in diagnosing people likely to develop Alzheimer's). I was amused by the frequent requests for money to import mice from Sweden.

I am sure that many QRD members take the whole thing very seriously and have much greater understanding of the science; nevertheless I hope that my rapid, at times rough and ready, assessments contributed something to the whole. And, as I mentioned, my comments were anonymous.

I resigned from the QRD panel in 2009 as I felt I was perhaps getting a little bitter and twisted with Margaret's continued deterioration.

2006

Care Changes

As 2005 drew to a close there had been some disquiet among the New Forest Homecare girls, because there were rumours of a substantial reorganisation of their duties. I couldn't help being aware of the mutterings, although nobody had breached any confidentiality. It became clear in 2006 that many of their present clients were to be passed to private companies. I was very happy with the care being provided for Margaret by the Social Services Homecare team and I made this clear; I was visited by the Manager, who assured me that her team would continue to care for a limited number of long term clients, including Margaret.

However the rumours persisted and strengthened. On March 20 2006 I phoned to seek further reassurance; but I was told that the previous assurances were no longer valid. Margaret's care would be transferred to a private care company. On March 31 I heard that a Care Manager had been appointed and would be in charge of the transfer arrangements.

Rhoda came to see us on April 3. I told her that I was worried about the possible unsettling affect on Margaret's health. At her suggestion I phoned the Service Manager, Adult Services, who was several rungs up the hierarchy ladder. I dictated a message which was transcribed efficiently by his PA and I received a letter in reply shortly afterwards, thanking me for the praise that I was heaping on the Department but asserting that the transfer was to go ahead.

I couldn't see any point in continuing discussion (why fight a war that can't be won?) so I decided to concentrate my efforts on making it all work

The Care Manager and Team Leader came for a meeting, for which I had prepared a written agenda; I also produced a detailed description of the care being provided for Margaret, and pointed out the need for carers with experience of Alzheimer's who would be able to cope with TIAs, fits and other disturbances, as well as providing continuity. This input was used as the basis for a written care plan, which was sent for my agreement and then used for negotiation with several agencies.

Willow Tree

It all turned out very well – in fact, brilliantly. Social Services placed a contract with Willow Tree Homecare Ltd (based in Lymington) a new, enthusiastic company formed the previous year, which was keen to expand its portfolio of clients. The Managers, Michaela and Janine, came for an initial meeting which went well. I was impressed by their businesslike approach.

Willow Tree Homecare Ltd took over Margaret's care on May 06 2006.

I am pleased to record that I was very satisfied with Willow Tree's performance from the start. Michaela left the company and an excellent relationship developed with Janine (who now owns the Company) and her team of managers and carers. They were all delightful people and the care they provided for Margaret could not be bettered. When I hear unhappy stories about other agencies, I believe that we were very fortunate and I am grateful to all those who contributed to the successful transfer.

Away days

Willow Tree operated sitting and sleep-over services in addition to their Personal Care activities. Margaret's condition stabilised as 2006 progressed and, with a clear conscience, I was happily able to arrange a day out on October 25. This was my first full day away for many years. Margaret was left in the capable hands of Tina, a carer who had access to Willow Tree for back-up if needed. I went by train to Clapham Junction where Christopher met me. He showed me his new flat in Battersea, then we joined Heather with Tom, Holly and Jo (my grandchildren) at the Zia Teresa an Italian restaurant that we'd frequented for many years. The sun was shining; it was a lovely day

Although I had twice-weekly two-hour breaks (leaving Margaret with Jennifer or sometimes another sitter from SCA), taking a whole day out and meeting the family was a wonderful relief from the stress of 24/7 care during Margaret's deterioration over several years. I found everything in order when I returned at 6.00pm; Tina had given Margaret her lunch (and clearly enjoyed her own which I had left ready) the girls had come and gone, Margaret was already in bed sleeping. I felt a new sense of liberty as I realised that I could repeat the experience.

Later Heather, Christopher and I met for a magnificent lunch at Westminster College, Vincent Square, where Chris had studied hotel management from 1976-78. Gemma, the young sister of Janine (and also a trained carer) looked after Margaret; again, all was well.

I have arranged away days several times each year ever since these first trials. I should make it clear that whereas the two weekly two hour sessions of sitting time, from which I have benefitted since 2001, are financed by Social Services, I pay for the support on my extra days privately. Typically each day is charged at over £100; so in times of decreasing resources and increasing cost of living, I try to ensure that my time away from the 24/7 job is well spent.

Hoist

In the last few months of 2006, helping Margaret to sit then stand up from bed in the morning was becoming very difficult. Often I would assist the carers so I knew that considerable physical effort was needed. Some of the girls were feeling strain in their backs.

Eventually Charlotte (a Student Nurse working with Willow Tree during her vacation) and Gemma, asked for my agreement to start using the hoist that we had stored since the end of 2005. They had both been trained in handling; the change was a great success. From this time on, the carers would clean Margaret on the bed, then hoist her into the glide-along chair ready for her shower (or, if needed, to sit in the chair over the WC).

Margaret has never complained about being hoisted – apparently this is fairly unusual. I can only suggest that it is because she was brought up within a short distance from Blackpool Pleasure Beach, where people pay hard-earned cash for similar experiences.

Thrush and other problems – well done the NHS

Margaret developed a rash in her groin. One of the district nurses, Karen, came to see Margaret. She thought the problem was thrush and went back to see the GP, who prescribed Canesten This was delivered by Lloyds and the problem cleared after ten days.

I must mention the excellent service provided over many years by Lloyds Pharmacy, Avenue Road, New Milton. They were very co-operative and always managed to pull out the stops if urgent action was requested.

A different rash in the groin was observed a few weeks later. Another GP came to see her; she suggested that the problem was due to rubbing by night pads soaked in urine, and prescribed Fucidin. This was quickly effective.

Another commendation! The GP Practice in New Milton was always very quick to respond and, if needed, to visit when I phoned about new problems.

During the night of September 22 Margaret had been very wheezy; I had rubbed her with Vick but the problem was worse by morning. The carers and I were concerned. It was a Saturday, so I phoned the emergency line. The response was impressive: I was asked to hold the telephone by Margaret's chest, so that the wheezing could be heard; and by 10.30 we were visited by the duty doctor who prescribed amoxycillin. Incredibly he carried bottles of granules that just had to be made up with boiled water. Margaret's treatment started within minutes.

The wheezing continued and I requested a follow up visit. One of our regular GPs sounded out Margaret and declared that her chest seemed clear; but the amoxicillin should continue until the end of the week. Happily by this time Margaret was breathing normally again.

Back to me

Early in 2006 I started to feel pain in my right knee. The doc thought that this was probably a strain which would go away; but it got worse and by August I was walking with a stick because I never knew when my knee was going to give way. It was suggested that an X-ray would be helpful in diagnosing the problem.

It turned out that several weeks would elapse before I could get an NHS appointment at Lymington Hospital and no definite time could be booked – which made it impossible to arrange a sitter without incurring vast expense.

However I have paid out shed-loads of money to AXA-PPP (formerly PPP) so that I could have private treatment when needed and I was able to get an immediate appointment at the Nuffield Hospital, Bournemouth. The doc gave me a referral note and on the following Wednesday, when Jennifer was sitting with Margaret, I drove to the Nuffield, had the X-ray, waited for the prints and brought them back with me; I left them at the surgery for attention. All this was achieved within the two hour limit of my time out.

I saw the doc, after he had heard back from the Nuffield. He told me that their report stated the problem was due to gout, resulting from crystals forming in the knee joint; there was calcified cartilage, but no sign or arthritis. He prescribed allopurinol, which I have been taking ever since.

But the swelling and pain in my knee continued. In the absence of my usual doc I made an appointment with another GP at the Practice, who I had already met several times. He suggested taking Mobic, an NSAID that I had used previously, but after several weeks it was clear that this didn't help.

I was also having trouble with my feet. Both big toenails had turned black. Lamisil, combined with an antibiotic, Flucloxacillin was prescribed. Later my blood pressure pills were changed to Ramipril and, as I was feeling rather ill, the Flucloxacillin was discontinued.

Rhoda came to visit Margaret; she was concerned about me, pointing out that my innards must by now be working like a chemical factory, and suggested that I needed a holiday.

By a curious and very fortunate coincidence one of the Willow Tree carers attending Margaret was Ginny (an ex-nurse) who told me that her husband had experienced a similar knee pain. He was referred to a consultant specialising in such problems, who had rapidly cured him by extracting fluid from his knee then giving a steroid injection.

2007

I was referred to this genius and on January 05, 2007, I went to see him at the Nuffield. I staggered into his consulting room with my stick in one hand and the X-rays (which I had retrieved from the GP's surgery) in the other.

The consultant said this was a classic case of pseudo-gout caused by an accumulation of calcium pyro-phosphate crystals in the knee – different from conventional gout which is caused by uric acid crystals usually in the foot joints. He offered to treat me on the spot and withdrew over 100ml of liquid from my knee, then gave me a steroid injection. I felt better almost immediately and was able to walk happily away from the Nuffield to my waiting taxi, without using my walking stick.

My knee problems had been depressing me for several months. My 24/7 caring job necessitates spending many hours a day on my feet; I had even been walking round the house with a stick for many weeks. Now I returned to my usual happy disposition overnight. Life has been much better ever since.

However, many years later I still take a folding walking stick with me if I am likely to be out for some time (for example on my away days). I keep another stick in the car, and I try to avoid twisting round suddenly, just in case. I go down stairs very slowly, always holding on to something.

This note about my health at this time is included as background to the problems I was experiencing in coping with Margaret's deterioration.

Royal blood?

At 10.25 on Saturday 3rd February 03, 2007 the carers Ginny and Samantha reported that both Margaret's hands had turned blue/purple. Her numbers were not good: I checked her BP at 171/164, with pulse 149. These emergencies often seem to happen on Saturdays. I phoned the NHS doctor's out-of-hours number, explained the situation, and at 12.10 a sister phoned back. I had continued monitoring BP, which by this time had returned to the more acceptable level 136/83.

The sister suggested that there might be some sort of mechanical problem caused by hoisting. Margaret stayed in bed all day and was fine on the next day. There was no sign of blue hands. I sent a report to the Practice.

Congestion

Margaret continued to wheeze regularly; I was dealing with this by administering amoxycillin, as prescribed the previous year. I needed a further supply and, as phone requests are not accepted, I left a note with the Practice receptionist, requesting a repeat prescription. I was phoned that evening by another doctor from the Practice, querying my request. I described Margaret's symptoms.

He suggested that the congestion was possibly caused by a build up of fluids, that could be cured by a diuretic. He prescribed liquid furosemide, which quickly cured the problem. I gave this medicine to Margaret whenever she started to wheeze – often during the night or on waking in the morning. It usually took about 20 minutes for the problem to clear. However I have now discontinued use of furosemide for Margaret because in later years the heavy urination seemed to be followed by an epileptic fit. I have never convinced a doctor about this observed link.

Further deterioration

Margaret had a major fit on Saturday April 07. The carers were helping her return to the bedroom after being showered and dressed, when she started shaking and sat down on the chair being pushed behind her. I was in the room and held her hand; her legs also started to shake; her eyes glazed over. We lifted her legs and, when the shaking subsided, put her back on the bed, where she slept until mid-afternoon, then woke and had an egg sandwich, my standard pick-me-up for her on these occasions. Although she seemed to be OK the next day, I suspect that this event was the start of a significant change.

During the week of April 23 there was obvious deterioration. Until this time Margaret had been feeding herself with a special spoon and plate that I had bought. But this capability just disappeared overnight. From then on, Margaret has had to be spoon and hand fed, with drinks in small glasses being held to her mouth.

On May 06, after a 'normal' day I said good night at 6.30. I looked in several times and at 7.30 she was fast asleep. But when I went to bed at 11.30 I found she had been sick. I cleaned her up as much as possible but she made no response.

On the following day I woke her as usual at about 9.00am. She accepted the drink of milk (mixed with metoclopramide and magnesium hydroxide, as usual) which I held to her mouth, but wouldn't take the small honey sandwich I had brought. Her face was very red, but her temperature was slightly under normal. The carers, Hyacinth and Chrissie, cleaned her up and left her in bed. They returned at lunchtime to change her; she didn't wake or respond while being changed.

I checked her BP several times during the day; it was 175/126, fell to 138/79, then rose again to 178/94. Different carers returned at 5.45. We were all concerned. Margaret's face and most of her body were bright red by this time. After discussion with Ginny I phoned NHS Direct. We didn't know whether Margaret might have had a stroke.

The duty doctor came at 20.05; he pushed and pummelled Margaret to check her reactions, although she hardly woke up. He thought it unlikely that Margaret had suffered from a stroke but that she had an infection which was causing the bright red colouration. This doctor, too, left amoxicillin for me to make up with boiled water.

By the next morning she was brighter and ate small pieces of bread with honey. The carers cleaned her in bed and she slept for most of the day. Her appetite had returned; BP was down to 130/74. Her breathing was bad, but seemed better after her doses of amoxicillin.

On Wednesday, 09 May, I gave her amoxicillin at 08.30 but couldn't wake her for breakfast at 09.15. I phoned to request a doctor's visit; a GP came at 12.20. He couldn't detect any fluid on her chest and suggested continuing with the one week course of antibiotic. On the next day Margaret was a lot better. We wheeled her to the lounge and hoisted her onto her reclining chair. Within a few days she was back to walking, with someone holding her hands and walking backwards to support her, and another carer following with a wheelchair.

Electric hoist

For some time Margaret had transferred to her wheelchair before lunch so that she could sit at the table with me. Sometimes I would then take her out in the wheelchair but if she looked tired after lunch I would transfer her to the reclining chair. I had been able to do this alone, helping her to stand then back her onto the recliner; but by now this was no longer possible as she was not able to put any effort into the transfer or even to comprehend what I was trying to do.

I decided to seek specialist handling advice but found that the Becton Centre OT was no longer doing outreach visits. I was referred to Social Services for help and was visited on Friday May 18 by an OT attached to Social

Services, who was new to the area and very enthusiastic. She suggested that the problem could be solved by having an electric hoist (which I could operate on my own) instead of the original manual hoist that was still being used.

This OT proved to be effective in getting things moving; an electric hoist was delivered on June 01. She returned a few days later to give me a short course on using the equipment, including fitting the sling to Margaret and attaching it to the hoist. I transferred Margaret several times; then the OT declared that she was satisfied that I could safely use the hoist on my own to transfer Margaret as needed. The electric hoist was welcomed by the carers; I realise that we have been very fortunate because I was told that ours was the only one they saw on their rounds; they were very scarce in the New Forest at that time.

The OT returned in July, accompanied by an expert on handling who specified a change in the sling being used; new padded types were delivered which have proved more comfortable for Margaret. She also arranged for the supply of an Oddstock Wedge, which was available to support Margaret's legs in bed, if needed.

No more walking!

Margaret took her last few steps on Friday May 25 2007. Hyacinth and Chrissie had showered her, then stood her to be dressed; but she went down on the floor. I called for an ambulance (this is standard procedure) which came within a few minutes. The paramedic and his assistant used a series of inflatable cushions to raise Margaret to a height from which they could slide her onto the glide-along chair; then the girls took her to the lounge and hoisted her onto her recliner.

Until this time the received wisdom had been that we must try to keep Margaret walking for as long as possible, even if only for a few steps. But I made an executive decision that this practice should cease and Margaret should be hoisted and wheeled for all movements. I soon realised that the effort of continuing to walk had been a great strain – physical and mental – on Margaret; within a few weeks she became a more tranquil, happier person.

Life remained fairly calm for the rest of 2007. We seemed to have established a harmonious regime; inputs and outputs were all working regularly; Margaret seemed happy and comfortable. Strain on the carers was reduced now that we had settled for hoisting and wheeling, without any attempt at standing or walking.

There were a few minor incidents – thrush, and a patch on Margaret's head were all cured with the help of the medical team.

Margaret and I had a quiet Christmas together, with carers coming and going as usual. Heather, Royston, Jo and Christopher all came to stay for New Year.

2008

Jaundice

The New Year started well then, on January 31, we noticed that Margaret was turning yellow. (We'd already seen her in blue and red; was this to be the 2008 fashion?)

I phoned the GP, who thought the symptoms sounded like jaundice and produced the remarkable information that Margaret had previously suffered from jaundice when she was 15. He said that there was no treatment, and that the condition would probably clear after a few days. It did.

By February 03 the colouration had gone and Margaret was OK again.

Fits (and misfits)

On Thursday March 06 Margaret had some sort of fit while the carers were cleaning her, before transfer to the shower chair. Her legs went up in the air, her arms were shaking and her eyes were rolling around. I checked her BP (138/78), temperature (97.1) and pulse rate (78), then phoned for a doctor who came at 10.30. She thought that this was a small fit, not a TIA.

We kept Margaret in bed; she slept all day but managed to munch an egg sandwich at 2.30, followed by a jam sandwich at 4.30; then after the girls washed and changed her, she settled her down to sleep at 5.30.

On the next day Margaret had a similar fit with waving legs and arms, and eyes rolling, when the carers were cleaning her on the bed. This time I was watching and noted that the problem started when they rolled her onto her right side. However, she soon recovered so they showered and dressed her as usual. For the next two days the carers minimised the time spent on her right side. Within a week the problem seemed to have cleared. There was no recurrence until 2010.

These incidents emphasise the care and observation needed when looking after an Alzheimer's patient, especially in the late stage. You never know what tomorrow will bring. If there is an event – is this something new? Or similar to a previous occurrence, which can be tackled with experience?

Kim

On April 8, 2008, Rhoda was here for her usual six-weekly visit. She had previously arranged to bring a mature student nurse, Kim, to see what life is like at the coalface. I gave a quick summary of the most significant events, then asked if she had any questions or comments.

"Yes," Kim replied. "Do you grieve?"

This was the first time in years that anyone had shown any interest in how I have felt and still feel about Margaret's illness. Kim's question touched me and I'm not ashamed to admit that I almost cried. But I didn't. That came later.

I later invited Kim to spend a day with us; she came at 8.00 on Monday 09 May. I encouraged her to do everything that I would normally do. I involved her immediately in giving Margaret her early milk and honey sandwich. Later she had a chat with the carers (Hyacinth and Chrissie) over coffee. During the morning Margaret slept and I talked with Kim about the advantages of keeping a patient at home instead of consigning her to a care home. Kim helped her with her medicine and orange drink before the carers came to change Margaret and transfer her to the wheelchair.

It was a lovely sunny day. We all had lunch outside. Kim fed Margaret and we continued our chat. Before she left I asked for her immediate reaction. She said that all her previous nursing experience had been in wards, where there is always someone senior to take responsibility when needed. But she had realised during the day that when an Alzheimer's patient continues to live at home, it is the 24/7 carer who takes full responsibility.

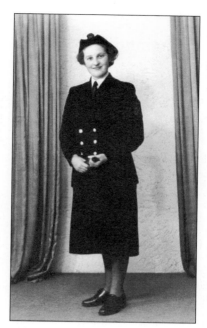

Petty Officer Wren Margaret Wood in 1952

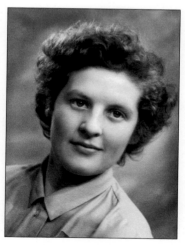

Margaret in 1952

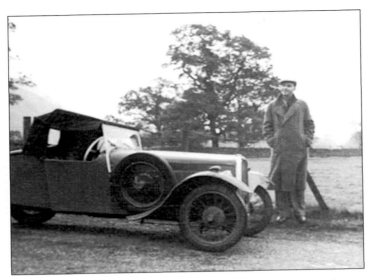

B.S.A. Threewheeler in the Lake District 1953

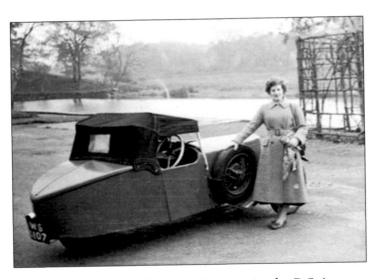

*Expedition to the Lake District in the B.S.A.
threewheeler, 1953*

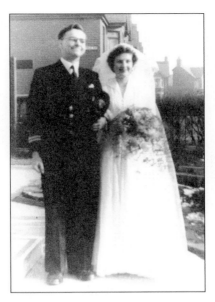

Our wedding in Blackpool, February 19th 1955

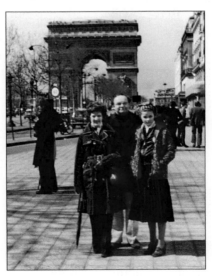

Paris with Heather in 1977

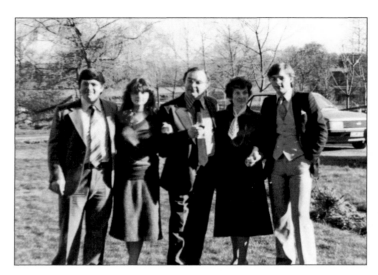

Silver Wedding 1980 at Wallingford

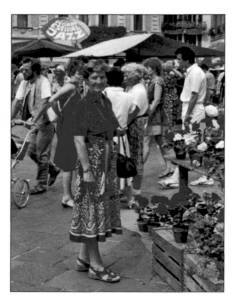

Lugano 1983 Jazz Festival time.

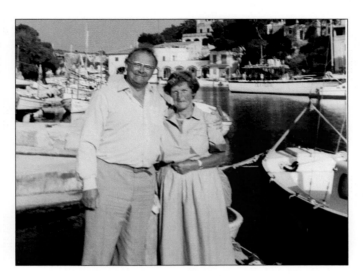

Mallorca 1987

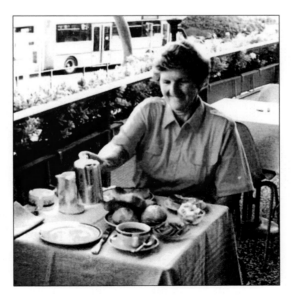

Breakfast in Geneva 1989

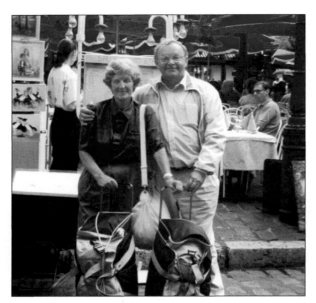

Paris 1991

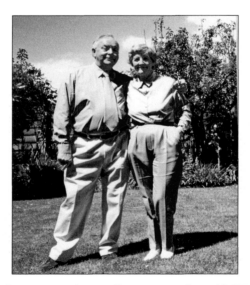

In our garden at Barton-on-Sea, 1997

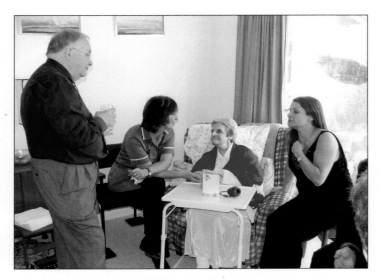

Golden Wedding 2005 with Heather and Sue Cooper

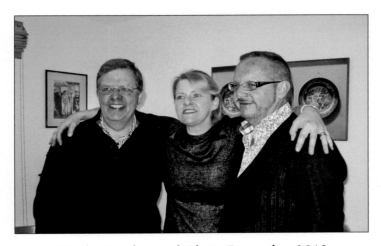

Mark, Heather and Chris, December 2012

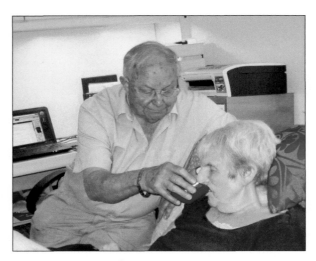

Caring for Margaret in 2013

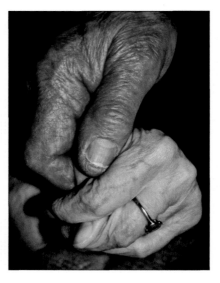

Together
(From a study by Rosie May Bird Smith)

Guests

Margaret was always very happy when we had guests. We used to have a pub lunch sometimes with Ruth and Ken. This had not been possible for several years, but we were often invited to Chez Stannard, across the road. I would trundle Margaret over in her wheel chair; Ruth made superb meals, which we both appreciated. Similarly I would invite Ruth and Ken over for lunch. We still managed to celebrate birthdays, anniversaries and feast days.

2009

UTIs and other problems

In the first few weeks of 2009 Margaret continued with the tranquil life that had developed by late 2008. But there were occasional perturbations.

On 26th February, 2009, Verity and Noi, the duty carers, reported a possible UTI (Urinary Tract Infection – a problem with Alzheimer's patients because there is a high risk that the infection will spread; this has been reported to be one of the main causes of death).

A five day course of trimethoprim was prescribed by phone, then by March 01 it seemed that the problem had cleared. On March 07 there was a brief reappearance of the discharge that had alerted the carers; by the next day all was clear again.

On March 16 Margaret awoke with severe wheezing and coughing, at 11.30pm. I gave her a dose of furosemide. At 07.30am I gave her a second dose, as the problem had continued and she was obviously in discomfort, and the discharge had reappeared.

One of the GPs came to see her and confirmed that Margaret had a chest and urinary infection. She prescribed a seven day course of co-amoxiclav.

By March 24 the discharge had stopped but the chest infection continued. Norzol (metronidazole) was prescribed by phone. But the discharge continued. I was increasingly concerned.

This time the visiting doctor prescribed amoxycillin to be used as standby. However the Norzol must have worked because the infection cleared and I had no need to open the amoxycillin.

Tom: – diabetes? Shock! Horror!

During March I was invited to have a blood test. The result showed a high sugar level and in May I attended a clinic with our GP and the Practice sister specialising in diabetes. I was urged to take strict measures to lose weight (at that time I was well over 15st.) and given dietary advice which I took very seriously. Amlodipene was added to my daily cocktail of pills, to reduce my blood pressure. My type 2 diabetes has so far been diet controlled; I attend for check-ups every six months.

It seems to me that type 2 diabetes is perhaps an occupational hazard for 24/7 carers (especially males). There is a strong urge to eat and drink in the evenings as compensation for stress and, above all, loneliness. This sometimes leads to obesity and then diabetes. I appeal to all the medicos – doctors, nurses, visiting carers – who attend Alzheimer's patients, please keep watch on 24/7 home carers who you encounter.

Take a Break

Early in 2009 the Government announced that money was being made available, through PCTs, which would enable home carers to have some respite. I followed this up but found that the money had not been ring-fenced and was being diverted by many PCTs to other uses. I understood that only 100 hours of breaks were available, in 2009, for the New Forest.

After the topic had been covered in a BBC report, I wrote to the Hampshire PCT. I was told that their extremely limited resources for respite care were being used to provide help for young carers looking after older people, with which I couldn't disagree. I concluded that the scheme was a political PR stunt and abandoned further action.

Changes at the Becton Centre

Rhoda Curtis, the CPN who had been my guide, consultant, friend and general guru since 2001, retired at the end of July. Her place was taken by Kim who had graduated and was happy to return to Barton.

Holiday in London

My first respite break since the onset of Margaret's Alzheimer's disease was from August 19 – 21, 2009. Two of the Willow Tree girls Kath (days) and Babs (nights) came to stay with Margaret; I met Heather and Royston in London and we all stayed at the Holiday Inn, Great Marlborough Street. The building was previously a famous Magistrates' Court, where Royston had been on duty many times during his career with the Met. We had a super time, with several excellent meals and enough (more than?) to drink. Christopher came in to join us. On the first night we went to Ronnie Scott's (something I'd wanted to do for a long time) then on the second night we went to the Palladium, round the corner, to see the musical *Sister Act*. By the time I returned home I felt I had been away for a month! And the girls had cared for Margaret with all their usual kindness; she was fine.

Carcinoma

During September 2009 a small spot appeared above Margaret's upper lip at the left side. Previously she had a wart that was treated with a cream; but this spot didn't respond. A doctor thought it might be a Basal cell carcinoma and advised the application of Fucidin while waiting to see what happened. The spot didn't go away.

On November 27 another doc advised further investigation and referred Margaret to the Dermatology Unit at Christchurch Hospital. After I explained the problems with transport logistics, a specialist from Christchurch came to our house on December 01 and did a biopsy.

Life trundled on – but the spot started to grow. Eventually on Dec 22 I was told that the results of the biopsy were inconclusive. A small committee had been considering the problem. I explained that this was academic and the spot – now a growth the size of a pea – had to be dealt with urgently. I emailed photos of the growth with a ruler alongside to the doc who had performed the biopsy.

Margaret was then referred to the Maxillofacial Surgery Unit at Poole Hospital. Thus she was in the system, at least.

The growth above Margaret's upper lip rapidly expanded. By early January 2010 it was 1.5cm across; in the next two weeks it grew another centimetre. After phone calls to Poole I found that the consultant would be away towards the end of January. I sent him a new set of photos. Margaret was admitted on January 21 and the carcinoma was removed the next day. A solar keratosis on her left upper leg was also removed. A flap of skin had been folded down from the side of Margaret's nose to seal the wound where the carcinoma had been removed. The histology report stated that there were no signs that the growth might spread (no vascular invasion), but I was warned to keep a watch, especially on her back as this would be the most likely site for any further problem.

The Maxillo Unit at Poole was brilliant. The surgeons were communicative and the nurses were all charming, efficient and caring. I stayed at a hotel in Poole for two nights.

On our return home Margaret's face was swollen and distorted, with 30-40 soluble stitches. Ruth and Jennifer gave massive support. Chris and Shaun came to see Margaret on the night we returned from Poole; Heather with Royston and George (the dog) visited a week later. They were all very upset.

I found it all a bit traumatic. Let's face it, I was shattered. But it's amazing how much one learns from these experiences – not least, about oneself.

On February 23 we returned to Poole for a follow up clinic with the consultant. He complimented himself on the excellent job he had done and said that no further visits would be needed unless new problems developed.

Our New Milton doctors and staff were very supportive as Margaret's condition improved and the wounds healed.

Visit to Heather

On Friday March 19 I visited Heather for a night while Babs from Willow Tree stayed with Margaret. I met Heather at the school where she was PA to the English Faculty, then we went off for a noggin with several of her friends before returning to her lovely home in Bromley. After a dinner of roast chicken (cooked by Tom) with Holly, Jo, Tom, Jenny and Royston we all had a very jolly evening which included an almost complete performance of *Oliver*. It was fun.

On my way home I realised how much we were missing by not living near to our family; I also decided that, after seeing Margaret's experience in Poole hospital, where she was immediately acclimatised, she would no longer miss our house in Barton-on-Sea. Before my train arrived at New Milton I had decided to sell our house and live, instead, in Bromley. It was time to move on.

In the next few days I talked with several estate agents, then appointed Ross Nicholas & Company who made a sale within a few weeks. I won't go into the attendant hassle, but there was a lot.

Intensive research by Heather and myself found three new flats in the Bromley area, which I visited at the end of May. On June 01 I visited the best of the three again and paid a deposit.

More UTIs

Meanwhile, back in Barton, the carers reported a heavy discharge on Friday 04 June. The Nurse Practitioner at the Practice visited her, took a swab, then prescribed Norzal. The discharge had cleared by the end of the six day course.

80!

While the removal was being planned I reached my 80th birthday. Heather had arranged a family lunch at Aldo Zilli's restaurant in Soho. On the night before I went with Chris and Shaun to a jazz bar in Battersea. Babs from Willow Tree again came to stay with Margaret overnight. It was a wonderful celebration!

Logistics

It was clear that no one involved would stick his or her neck out on the timing for the legal work to complete our property sale and purchase. So I instructed everyone that completion date would be August 10 (during Heather's school holiday).

Our Care Manager liaised with Bromley Adult Services and transmitted an updated assessment which was accepted without question. She also arranged for Margaret to spend a week in a Bromley Nursing Home during the removal in August.

The new Care Manager in Bromley was very helpful and welcoming. She placed contracts with SureCare Bromley for PC and with Bromley Mind for the Sitting Service.

On July 21st I had a day in Bromley, starting with a visit to the new flat to meet the developer and confirm arrangements for conversion of the bathroom to a walk-in shower room. The Risk Assessment Officer with Bromley Adult Services also came to see the flat and agree the equipment we would need. Then I went on to visit SureCare and finished at the Nursing Home where I briefed staff on the care that Margaret would need.

Lymington Hospital

Margaret awoke on Saturday 10 July with a stiff and swollen left leg. A doctor from the out-of-hours service arranged for her to be admitted to Lymington Hospital, because there might be a DVT (deep vein thrombosis). The Hospital and staff were all excellent and happily the scan found no trace of a DVT. Margaret came home on Tuesday 13 July. Her stiff, bent, leg has persisted; now both legs are bent. But the swelling has gone down. The medicos have no explanation. We just try to make sure she is comfortable.

Ready to Go!

While all this was happening I was busy downsizing. An amazing amount of furniture, paperwork from my business, books and other items had to be ditched. Many charity shops benefitted, if that's the right word.

Margaret moves to Bromley

I had booked a private ambulance to take Margaret to the Nursing Home in Bromley, on Saturday August 07. I also arranged with Willow Tree for Linda – an experienced carer (and ex-nurse) who knew Margaret well – to escort her and hand over to the staff.

Removal

The day arrived! Heather (with Royston) and Christopher offered magnificent support before, during and after the removal. Chris came to Barton and fortunately persuaded me to ditch a lot of stuff I had intended to bring. He was absolutely right. We filled 15 dustbin bags to leave behind. Chris and I stayed at the Cliff House Hotel, Barton, on Sunday August 08 and Monday 09 while the removal people cleared the house. The planning paid off. Despite many last minute traumas in the chain of purchasers, we succeeded in completing on August 10. Chris drove me to Bromley; he thought I might be too emotional to drive myself. While we were on the M25 I had a phone call saying that the completion had taken place and the keys of our new flat could be collected.

And that was the end of our 28 years living in Barton-on-Sea. Although we had been very happy there before Margaret's illness, I was becoming increasingly sad and lonely. Every time I went to the town or for a walk on the clifftop, I sensed the presence of Margaret alongside me. And there was no-one to talk with about my feelings, so they were bottled up, repressed. Not good! It had been time to go.

Life in Bromley, August 2010 onwards

Life in Bromley, August 2010 onwards

Heather collected the keys on completion and was waiting at the flat on August 10 after Chris had driven me over. She had stocked the cupboards and fridge – terrific! Heather sorted out many arrangements in Bromley with introductions to doctors, cleaning services, hairdressers, sitting services, and other indispensables.

I stayed with Heather on August 10 then the removal van came on the next day. Heather and Royston both helped enormously with the sheer effort of moving in. Margaret came out of the Nursing Home on Saturday 14 August, and the excellent service from SureCare started at lunchtime. Sarah and Sharon were the first carers to arrive.

Chaos and calm

The next few months were chaotic. We lived out of boxes, while I gave away much of the furniture that was brought from Barton and had new units designed, built and installed by Spacemaker Ltd in the lounge and front bedroom. Eventually we were more or less straight by mid-November.

Margaret stayed calm throughout all the comings and goings, accepting the new surroundings, routines and carers.

Pressure

Soon after we moved to Bromley, Sarah, then the carers' Team Leader, noticed a discolouration on the side of

Margaret's right heel. I phoned for help from a district nurse who came within hours and applied a dressing. We don't know how the problem happened. But soon the discolouration developed into an open wound or ulcer and another appeared on the opposite foot. The district nurses team came twice a week for several weeks before the wounds eventually healed. Margaret was not able to spend her afternoons in the wheelchair while the problem persisted, so I couldn't take her out for an afternoon walk as at Barton.

HomeCare Bromley

I am pleased with HomeCare Bromley (previously SureCare Bromley). The carers are well trained and punctilious; Margaret is well looked after. Many of the girls who come here are from Sri Lanka and I have found out a lot about their country. We also have carers from Ruanda, Bangladesh, Nepal, the Gambia, the Ivory Coast and elsewhere. Only a few of the girls are from the UK. Several girls have trained as nurses in their own countries but work as carers here, often combined with study for higher qualifications. Others are studying business administration, IT, accountancy and various different subjects; they are here on student visas. Our flat is now a *de facto* centre for international and inter-faith understanding. I like it!

Fits again

In November I went out briefly, to our local shops while Surangi and Sashikala were working through Margaret's getting up procedure. Surangi phoned me while I was waiting to pay and I returned asap. After her shower Margaret had started to shake; the SureCare girls had managed to get her back onto the bed and Surangi, who has many years' nursing experience back in Sri Lanka, correctly turned her onto her side.

The attack – later recognised as possibly a *grand mal* seizure– lasted about 5-6 minutes. It was all over by the time I returned – but I'd seen it before so I knew the symptoms and phoned for a doctor to come and check Margaret, the procedure established back in Barton. A doctor from the surgery in Bromley where we had registered came. This was our first contact. We discussed Margaret's condition and history. With my agreement he referred Margaret to a consultant physician for elderly people, to seek advice on the use of anti-epileptic medication. Margaret stayed in bed for the day and there were no signs of ongoing problems.

Bromley Healthcare, Long Term Conditions

(Previously NHS Care Coordination Team for Older People.)

During our discussion I had told the doctor that support, guidance and advice in the nursing and care for Margaret would be helpful, explaining that this had been provided previously by Rhoda Curtis, the CPN in the New Forest. A few weeks later I had the pleasure of an introductory visit by two nurses from the NHS Care Coordination Team for Older People which then provided a first contact/support point for carers who, like me, encounter difficulties and problems, or who need referring to another organisation. I am now visited every few weeks by the Community Matron who checks Margaret and discusses my concerns – to make sure that I am still coping. She liaises regularly with the Doctors' Practice. This care – for me! – is wonderful! A new experience!

Friendship

In November I met another denizen of the flats where we live in Bromley. Walking through the car park on my way back from the rubbish bins, one night in October, and feeling very lonely, I noticed that the interior light was on in a small Mercedes. The owner was on the phone and didn't hear my knock so I left a note under the door. Soon afterwards Joy came to thank me. This led to a splendid friendship. A few weeks later, over a dinner that I had cooked, Joy explained some of her plans for writing a book and starting a business. Since then my past industrial and writing experiences have helped Joy to start realising her ambitions. And I have found an outlet that is away from Alzheimer's.

2011

Another fit

Margaret had another fit at 09.40 on January 08. Again I was out; again the fit happened after Margaret's shower; again the very excellent Surangi looked after her. I had given Margaret a dose of furosemide at 03.30 as she was wheezing heavily. I don't know for certain that this led to the attack, but I believe there's a link

Eventually an emergency doctor came to see Margaret at 17.10. He sent a report to our GP in Bromley, whom I phoned to chase the referral made a few weeks earlier. We went by ambulance to see the consultant on February 07. After a very helpful discussion it was agreed that anti-epileptic drugs would not be a good idea because Margaret's resultant increased drowsiness would reduce her enjoyment of food, her only apparent remaining pleasure.

More sores

The district nurses came back because Margaret had a pressure sore. Obviously she is susceptible to this problem. An air mattress was installed, and there have been no more pressure sores.

Celebrations

We had our 56th anniversary on February 19, then celebrated Margaret's 80th birthday on March 13, with a small family party. Heather brought an excellent buffet; all her family came as well as Juanita and Michelle (Royston's mother and sister) and Joy. The lounge was full of flowers and cards.

Respite – Bromley Mind

Bromley Mind provides a sitting service for four hours each week enabling me to escape for shopping, banking, dentistry etc. I now have a six hour break every two weeks, with two hours in the intervening weeks. This is part of Margaret's care package.

Respite – Carers Bromley

A Respite Service provided by Carers Bromley enabled me to visit Boston, Lincolnshire, for two nights in March, to see Mark, Marian and their family. Timothy (trumpet) Matthew (sax) and I (keyboard) made great music, then on the next day we went to a wonderful gala concert with over 100 musicians from the Boston schools (Matthew and Tim both playing). It was a superb and memorable evening.

Carers Bromley also provide a subsidised sitting service that, for me, supplements the service from Bromley Mind.

Harina & Co. Ltd.

Planning for Joy's company was going ahead. We formed Harina & Co. Ltd. in June 2011. My main practical contribution was in helping to source products, where my industrial experience has been useful. We visited several companies, including some on a four day visit to Scotland in May 2011 to assess several cashmere manufacturers. SureCare arranged for a carer to stay here while I was away.

Harina: the Special Girl

Joy and I have written a childrens' book, based on a story that she has been thinking about for many years. We visited several publishers and talked with many more, but eventually decided to form our own publishing company, Harina & Co. (Publications) Ltd.

Our first book, *Harina: the Special Girl*, was published early in 2013. We have plans for several more in our *Tales of Harina* series. I mention these interests to emphasise how important it is to have a wide range of activities that occupy my mind, away from the caring job.

Painting holiday

In August 2011 I went for a short painting holiday in Whitstable, staying with Stephanie Brunton and Colin Whitaker whose house includes a large art studio and a music room. With three others I wandered round the quay looking for painting ideas, then Colin helped us to develop our talents. Three days of concentrated painting cleared my mind brilliantly – and hanging on the wall at home is my version of Whitstable quay to prove it. On the last night Stephanie (cello) Colin (guitar and double bass) and I (piano) made music. It was great!

Dementia UK and Admiral Nurses

While still living in Barton I had heard on the TV about Admiral Nurses, who provide long term support and advice to family carers looking after dementia sufferers. Admiral Nurses (all experienced mental nurses) are part of the charity Dementia UK, which also operates Uniting Carers, a nationwide network of family carers. As well as providing practical help and training, Dementia UK promotes the interest of family carers, by providing a voice that can make a difference in the services available, and increasing the national awareness of dementia.

I found that there were no Admiral Nurses working in either the New Forest area or Bromley – the number of nurses and their coverage is limited by the funds available, so I have had no personal experience of their work and support. However, a few years ago I filled in a form saying that I was willing to help promote the charity in its media work – articles, talks, interviews and other outlets.

Nothing happened until the autumn of 2011 when I received a phone call asking if I was still interested. The outcome was an invitation to attend media training sessions at the London HQ. These were enjoyable and stimulating – and led to a surprising development. I was asked to speak on behalf of Dementia UK at the opening of the 2011 Dementia UK Congress in November, in Liverpool. My talk and those from three other lay speakers can be found by entering 'Tom Wearden' on Google. The text is reproduced later in this book.

My seven minute slot, part of the plenary session, was attended by Paul Burstow who was then the Minister for Care Services. The audience numbered about 600 and included doctors, consultants, research workers, care managers, nurses and many other people with a professional interest in dementia. My talk was well received and I admit that it was a great ego-trip – finding that in my eighties I could still hold an audience did wonders for me.

2012

Continued tranquility

Margaret was very tranquil during 2012. The girls from SureCare came and went; they seemed happy, Margaret seemed happy. She had two small fits, both while the carers were helping with her morning ablutions, and stayed sleeping in bed for the day instead of being moved to the lounge.

Equipment

We had been using the wheelchair brought from Barton; ownership was transferred to the Wheelchair Service in Bromley. By this stage it was unsuitable to take Margaret out for walks, or to sit outside, because the back was upright and she had become so bent that she was not comfortable. After re-assessment by the Bromley Wheelchair Service in 2011 a new chair with partially sloping back was eventually delivered early in 2012. This was much more comfortable for moving around the flat. I tried leaving her in the wheelchair after the lunchtime carers' visit, then wheeling her outside for lunch. But this didn't work. Margaret by this time is so bent that I can't sit her up with her head in a comfortable eating position without hurting her neck.

We had also negotiated for the supply of a new shower chair, again with a sloping back. Unfortunately a wheel came off after a few months use. Getting a replacement took several weeks of negotiation.

Respite with party, painting and trains

I had several short breaks in 2012. My remaining brother-in-law, John (married to Margaret's younger sister, Rita) celebrated his 90th birthday in March with a family party in a hotel near Skipton, owned by friends. About thirty friends and family gathered during the day then sat down to a splendid dinner. Although disabled and severely disfigured after many facial operations, John made a good speech and I managed to say a few words of thanks on behalf of the guests (I never lose an opportunity!) We all stayed the night and I came home the next day. I like train travel and thoroughly enjoyed the journeys there and back.

Another train journey was to Torquay where I enjoyed a painting holiday with a group of 11 and an excellent tutor; we concentrated on painting water scenes in acrylic. Later in the year I journeyed to Devon by train again, this time to Hartland on the North coast for another few days' painting.

Finally, Joy and I had two journeys to York where we visited York Publishing Services Ltd and arranged for production of *Harina: the Special Girl*. (YPS has also produced the book you are now reading.)

So 2012 was a good year for 'respite'.

Move by Heather

I moved us to Bromley mainly to be nearer to Heather, our daughter. We met regularly for lunch on my days off. But, in October 2012, she and Royston went to live in Greenhithe, about an hour away, where they bought an attractive new house. They are happy. I still see them and it's always good to know they are not too far away. We still meet regularly in Greenhithe or Bromley.

The Conclusion.

Life continued steadily in Bromley until, in June 2014, I was diagnosed with 'wet' AMD (Age Related Macular Degeneration) in the right eye, which was treated with three injections of Eyelea (not fun). I could no longer drive.

Then, in October 2014, Margaret developed a rash, with large blisters on her back, arms and legs, diagnosed as Bullous Pemphigoid. The condition was thought to result from a failure in her immune system, which I believe was caused by her Alzheimer's disease. She was referred to the PRUH (Princess Royal University Hospital) in Farnborough, Bromley for treatment. After several days she came home with a pile of new pills, as well as instructions from the dermatologist that her blisters should be pierced with a sterile needle, drained and left to dry before applying dressings. I learned a new skill!

But it was all a bit too much for me. By December 2014 I too was in the PRUH, with a heart condition, Atrial Fibrillation.

With nobody at home to look after Margaret she was sent back to the PRUH. For some days, before being moved to our wards, we were both in the A&E Department.

After I was discharged, Heather and I set about finding a nursing home for Margaret because it was deemed too much strain for me to continue looking after her at home. With the help of the PRUH Margaret was moved on December 19th to the St. Aubyn's Nursing Home, Sidcup.

Margaret died from pneumonia on December 30th 2014. Her ashes now rest in the Garden of Remembrance, Christchurch Priory, where we worshipped together for many years.

A year later I decided to leave Bromley. Since July 2016 I have lived happily in a lovely, bright flat overlooking the sea at Hythe, Kent.

Tom Wearden   January 2017

Thoughts

Thoughts

Several years have passed since Margaret and I had a meaningful conversation, or exchanged a joke. Most of all I miss the fun and laughter we enjoyed together, ever since we first met. The daily grind continues, with occasional perturbations. Meals take a long time; Margaret eats well but slowly and of course she has to be spoon-fed all the time, which takes me 2-3 hours each day. I talk to her, telling her what I am doing, what we are having for lunch and other things. Margaret was always very fastidious about personal cleanliness and dressed well. I make sure that clean clothes, towels and bedding are always available for use by the visiting carers. Everyday is washday.

I'm sure that Margaret understands a great deal of the life around her. I believe that she knows when I am in the room. When someone is here having a chat with me she waggles her feet and sometimes even opens her eyes. No professional has attempted to estimate Margaret's level of consciousness; it could be part of an interesting research study. However, it seems that the Glasgow Coma Scale (GCS) is widely used and, looking at the definitions for Eye, Voice and Motor, the three elements, I would rate her as about 10 or 11 on a scale from 3 to 15. (Please see Wikipedia for comprehensive information about GCS and other systems for measurement.)

Life as a 24/7 carer for someone with Margaret's level of disability can be very lonely. I have few friends and, apart from our neighbour, Joy, none is local. There are no real opportunities to make new friends as going out is not simple; caring arrangements are essential – and expensive. Margaret is usually tucked up in bed before 6.pm. Evenings can be devastating, unless I plan some activity to keep me occupied. Overeating and drinking are occupational hazards. Just watching TV isn't enough – I like to be doing something at the same time, unless a gripping drama or discussion keeps me awake. Margaret used to love TV but has shown no interest or reaction for many years.

I see the carers every day and usually we have a few minutes for a short chat which is something of a lifeline. On days when they give Margaret a shower I have time for a short walk, or a visit to our local express store. The Pastoral Assistant from the local church brings communion every few weeks; there is usually time for a brief chat. Fortunately Joy and I meet several times each week; I remain very busy helping her with her new business, Harina & Co. Ltd., which keeps my brain ticking over as we tackle many challenging problems.

I look forward to the rare visits from our family, but I appreciate that they are sad to see their Mum as she is. However, we talk on the phone and they all seem to be enjoying their lives in different ways. I have often pondered that we are not here to run our children's lives – the most we can hope for is to equip them to run their own lives effectively. Seeing their progress, I feel that Margaret and I would be justified in finding a mild glow of satisfaction at a job reasonably well done, as I tell her from time to time.

So – how do I feel? Yes, Kim, even now I still grieve, for some part of each day. My route to survival involves keeping busy at all times. This is not too difficult. I write, I paint, I deal with paperwork; I enjoy cooking and preparing meals, I play jazzy improvisations on my clavinova.

And my life has been enriched by the experience of looking after Margaret for so many years, by the learning curve, by the new skills and understanding that I have acquired, by the happy relationship that I have with so many members of the caring community, and by the satisfaction that I feel when I see Margaret smiling, uncomplaining, still looking happy and well. The events and sometimes traumas associated with long term care of an Alzheimer's sufferer continue. But, as I have reminded myself for so many years, problems for others are challenges for us engineers. Margaret looked after me through our ups and downs for many, many years. Now it's pay-back time, and looking after her is an enriching privilege.

Margaret and I have shared a wonderful life together for 58 years. We have a super family: one daughter, two sons and six grandchildren. It is over ten years since we had any meaningful conversation. By now she is almost totally incapable; sometimes I talk with her about our life together and tell her we can look back and see that our early ambitions have been fulfilled. But for Margaret there is no past and no future – only the present, which changes with every second.

Finally, I never forget Margaret's advice from our first date in 1952:

'Food comes first' and
'Live every day as though it is the last'.

And so life continues along its merry way.
Tomorrow? Who knows?

Tom Wearden
Bromley, 2013

Life before Alzheimer's – the prequels

Life before Alzheimer's – the prequels

Margaret's story

Margaret Louisa Wood was born on 13th March 1931 at Preston Lancashire, the fourth of five sisters (Joyce, Nancy, Evelyn, Margaret and Rita). The family moved to Westgate Road, South Shore, Blackpool where Margaret lived for most of her childhood. On leaving school Margaret started work in a stockbroker's office. She studied shorthand, typing and other subjects at night school.

The Second World War had started in 1939, when Margaret was 8, and finished in 1945 when she was 14. The Wood family were heavily involved. Margaret's father, Frank Wood (known by all his family as Pop) was a hero of the First World War, in which he was commissioned as an officer in the Machine Gun Corps and won the MC. After the war he entered the insurance business. When I first met Pop he was an Area Manager with an office in Preston.

When the Second World War started Pop became a Special Constable, serving from 1939-1945. Margaret's mother, Emily (known to the family as Til), was engaged in helping families evacuated to Blackpool, and spent a lot of time looking after British, American and Australian members of the armed forces based in Blackpool who were often brought home by Margaret's older sisters. Joyce, her eldest sister joined the WAAF; her husband served in the RAF. Nancy was in the Auxiliary Fire Service; her husband

Ken also served in the RAF. Evelyn's husband, also Ken, served as an officer with the Royal Navy.

It was not surprising that in 1949, when she was 18, Margaret decided to join the WRNS (Women's Royal Naval Service, known as the Wrens) where her secretarial experience qualified for admission as a Writer in the Supply and Secretariat Branch. After training at HMS *Ceres* in Yorkshire she was posted to HMS *Excellent*, Portsmouth then to HMS *Cochrane*, Dunfermline.

However Margaret decided that life would be more exciting if she transferred to the Regulating Branch (the Naval equivalent to Military Police) and was accepted for training on a course that would lead to promotion as a Regulating Petty Officer. After experience back in Portsmouth (where she joined the WRNS Whaler Racing Crew which sailed in the Cowes Regatta) and at RNAS Culdrose, Margaret gained her PO's buttons in 1952. She was appointed to HMS *Sanderling*, a Royal Naval Air Station at Abbotsinch, near Paisley, Scotland. The site is now Glasgow Airport.

Tom's story

I was born in Didsbury, Manchester, apparently during a thunderstorm, on 22nd June 1930, the only son of May and Bertram Wearden. The family lived in Bramhall, Cheshire then moved to Wilmslow, Cheshire in 1934.

My father, Bertram Wearden, was a manufacturer's agent, specialisng in domestic hollowware. In the 1930s he had an office an showroom overlooking Piccadilly Gardens in the centre of Manchester. Sometimes when I was a small boy I would spend a day with him during school holidays. I gazed out of the window at the continuous movement of double decker tramcars, arriving from and setting off to all directions, mingling with cars, lorries and occasional horse-drawn trucks laden with bales of cotton. Perhaps it was the complex network of overhead cables, enabling the trams to move, which first stimulated my interest in electricity.

When war came in 1939 my father closed his office in Manchester and worked from home in Wilmslow, Cheshire. From 1938-1948 I attended Cheadle Hulme School (Manchester Warehousemen and Clerks' School) where I was 'on the science side'. In 1947-48, I was Head Boy. Both at school and in Wilmslow I was heavily involved in various drama activities, but I was aiming at a career in electrical engineering and in 1948 I won the Edmund Mills Harwood Scholarship to Manchester University, Faculty of Technology. I graduated BScTech in Electrical Engineering in 1951, having served as Vice President of the Students' Union from 1950-51. While at university I continued to be active in drama, producing many plays and shows as well as acting.

From 1951-1953 I served with the Royal Navy as a Sub Lieutenant (L) RNVR. I specialised in Fleet Air Arm electronic equipment and after training was appointed to HMS *Sanderling*, a naval airfield at Abbotsinch, near Paisley, where I was responsible for some 50 staff working on airborne and ground radio and radar installation and maintenance.

Together

It was at Abbotsinch that I met Margaret, who by then was a PO (Petty Officer) in the Regulating Branch of the WRNS. Margaret had joined HMS *Sanderling* towards the end of 1952. The first time Margaret saw me, I was on stage, dressed as a cat, in a pantomime that I wrote and produced. The first time I saw Margaret was on the following day when we were both singing in the chapel choir. She turned round and smiled at me. (Margaret later said she wondered what the cat's voice looked like in real life.) From that moment I never looked back.

Margaret has always been wonderfully good fun. On our first date she told me that she has two mottos: 'Food comes first' and 'Live every day as though it is the last'. Nothing changed. We never stopped finding things that make us both laugh, until her Alzheimer's came along.

In the first few months of 1953 we spent many happy hours together exploring different parts of Scotland whenever we could get away from the Air Station. It was at the Coronation Ball that we found we both liked dancing, and moved well together. We started as friends, but while we were still in the Navy, our developing love affair had to be treated with discretion. It survived!

Margaret was demobbed in the middle of 1953. She returned to live with her family and became secretary to the Planning Manager of Hawker Aircraft, a factory sited at Squires Gate Airfield, Blackpool, near to the family home.

After Margaret left HMS *Sanderling* I occupied myself by buying and re-building a run-down 1934 BSA three-wheeler car; then a colleague – one of the engineering officers – taught me to drive. Eventually I passed the RN driving test, on a three-ton truck.

I was demobbed in October 1953 at the end of my two years of National Service. However, I enjoyed naval life and remained a reserve officer for a further ten years, until work commitments became too heavy to continue. By this time I was a Lieutenant Commander (L) RNR.

While on demob leave I drove my BSA to Blackpool, to take Margaret away for a few days' holiday together. Her father came out to the road, kicked the car, and said: "You're not taking my daughter away in that thing are you? Is it insured?" Many years later I remembered this incident when our daughter Heather brought various boys home to meet the family.

After demob I joined Ferranti, Edinburgh, as a sales engineer based in London, responsible for their business in small transformers and microwave test equipment. I lived in Maidenhead. I had use of company car, so I sold the three-wheeler and later bought an engagement ring which resulted in t'wedding o' t'year on February 19 1955, at St Mary's, South Shore, Blackpool. We honeymooned in the Cotswolds, which were covered by deep snow.

We were very hard up! We lived in flats at Claygate and then Esher in Surrey. In 1956 I transferred to the Computer Department of Ferranti in London, to gain development engineering experience. Margaret was a secretary with an engineering consultancy company, Merz and McLellan, then with Pan Books. We lived off my salary and banked Margaret's, so that we could save for the deposit on a house, then in 1956 we managed to buy our first property, in Maidenhead. Unexpectedly my job was moved from London to Bracknell. We had no car, as I wasn't then concerned with sales, so I cycled ten miles to work each day. Not pleasant! Our first son, Mark Thomas, was born at home in Maidenhead in April 1957.

In 1959 I escaped from my cycling purgatory. I joined Vactric Control Equipment, London, as a sales engineer based in the Midlands, looking after sales of servo motors and various other electro-mechanical devices. We moved to Sutton Coldfield, Warwickshire. Here our next son,

Christopher John, was born in February 1960, also at home, followed by our daughter Heather Margaret in January 1963, at home again, this time in thick snow. I almost gained my certificate, as the midwife arrived only ten minutes before the birth. Margaret's mother came to stay with us on each occasion to look after Margaret when I had to return to work. However when Heather was born both boys developed measles and, of course, Margaret was in bed, so I had a mini-hospital to run.

In 1963 we moved to Marlow, Buckinghamshire. I had joined a French electronics company to set up a British subsidiary, marketing electronic components. We were based in Slough to be near Heathrow Airport. I travelled a lot and, as this was a great company for meetings, I was over in Paris every few weeks. As soon as our three children were all at school Margaret became a nursery school teacher – work that she greatly enjoyed. She did a part time course and qualified. Margaret has always loved little children and was never happier than when making them laugh.

In 1971 we moved to Melbourn, a village ten miles south of Cambridge, where I managed a materials science company specialising in crystal growth and associated equipment. Heather went to a local school and the two boys travelled into Cambridge where they were educated at the Cambridge High School for Boys. Margaret was active in village and church social life, and made many friends. We joined a jazz club and had many happy evenings listening and dancing to well known bands.

Our next move, to Bromley, Kent, was in 1976. I joined Lee Green Precision Industries, Blackheath, as commercial director in 1976. We became involved in the new, expanding fibre optics communications industry. Margaret worked at the Army and Navy Stores, Bromley, part of the House of Fraser Group. She enjoyed life in a big store and, as she has always had impeccable taste for clothes, found an outlet for her talents in the Separates Department. Both boys had left school; Mark was starting a career in banking and Chris went to Westminster Hotel School. Heather continued her education at the Baston School, Hayes.

When I reached 50, in 1980, I decided to put up a notional brass plate and call myself a consultant.

Mark and Chris had by this time left the nest and Heather had finished with school. We moved to Wallingford where we had a riverside house and a small boat. This meant we were nearer to Marlow, where my aging widowed mother lived. After her death in 1981 we moved in 1982 to Barton-on-Sea, fulfilling a long held wish to live by the sea.

I found that there was a good market for articles in technical magazines and started to write extensively for *Electronics Times*, *Electronic Engineering*, *Design Engineering*, *Automotive Engineering* and many other publications. In the next few years I produced over 500 feature articles which, combined with a growing management consultancy Practice specialising in fibre optics and other high-tech products, enabled us to live happily.

The operating principle of my consultancy work – like many consultancies, perhaps most – was summarised in the well known quotation ascribed to Desiderius Erasmus of Rotterdam (1466-1536):

'In the country of the blind, the one-eyed man is king.'
Guidance for my writing activity was provided by Dr Johnson:

'No man but a blockhead ever wrote, except for money.'

Margaret read everything I wrote. She was always particularly good at checking to make sure that I don't make too many mistakes in life. We often travelled together on working visits and had some excellent holidays during this time.

In 1997, when we were both 67, I abandoned the unequal struggle and 'retired'. Margaret had been in hospital for stomach ulcers (1987) hysterectomy (1987) and varicose veins (1995). I had cataract ops on both eyes (1993, 1996). Margaret was starting to show the first signs of her future problems; she increasingly needed help, support and, most important, TLC. I gradually took over the household jobs and within a few years she was diagnosed with Alzheimer's disease. Soon Margaret depended on me as her full time carer.

And that's how I moved into my next profession.......

Coping with Caring at Home

Coping with Caring at Home

Adapted from Tom Wearden's talk to some 600 professionals attending the Dementia UK Congress, 2011, in the presence of Paul Burstow MP, at that time Minister of State for Care Services.
The talk can be seen at http://vimeo.com/38085132 "

In 1970 Margaret looked at me, sadly, after her mother's funeral. She said:

'Please, promise you won't send *me* away to die like that, if I get Alzheimer's.'

We saw her mother, who'd had Alzheimer's for several years, a week before she died, in a ghastly mental hospital, where she'd been sent after her husband wasn't able to manage any longer at home. Her lovely curly hair had been cut very short. Many patients in the ward were partially dressed, shouting, pleading for help.

After seeing her mother's deterioration from being a wonderful, lively, bright-eyed caring lady, Margaret often spoke about her own fear of Alzheimer's. And she had nightmares, as well

In 1998, 28 years later, my lovely wife showed the first signs. Early in 2001 she, too, was diagnosed with Alzheimer's.

I'm Tom, 81. I've cared for Margaret at home for 13 years. It's not the retirement with fun and travel that we'd both hoped for. But I've found some compensation.

This is my experience of long term care at home.

My personal strategy, from the early days 13 years ago, has been to separate her care, my 24/7 job, from the sustained grief that underlies my emotions.

So far I've kept the promise I made to Margaret, 41 years ago.

Since 2004 over 250 visiting carers have looked after her personal care. These carers have been my main social contact for many years. They keep me cheerful! The perks of this, my fourth profession, include regular visits by beautiful, smiling girls in uniform!

In 2010 we moved to Bromley, Kent. Our visiting carers here are excellent SureCare girls, from many different countries. We have regular visits from the Community Matron, also from a highly spectacular tall blond voluptuous nurse, who wears a pleasantly short skirt. She gives me a hug then takes my blood pressure. For some reason it's always high!

(Unfortunately this lovely nurse and her family have now moved away).

So, 'coping' – with what?

As a professional engineer I'm a tactile, 'hands-on' person. I'm not afraid of involvement in the shirt sleeves and rubber gloves stuff. We engineers like to see problems as challenges, and sometimes we even invent solutions.

Earlier, on my own, there was a lot of handling, as Margaret's ability for purposeful movement faded; and there was toileting and washing as she lost control of her bowel actions.

Fortunately nowadays our visiting carers look after most of her personal care. But every day is washday; and there's still hand feeding – which takes me 2-3 hours a day. There's still handling, too, as I adjust her position in bed and on her chair.

All these tasks were increasingly difficult as Margaret's personality changed. From being a happy, feisty, fun-loving girl, an ex-Wren, always a joy to be with, always laughter, always humour, always taking the mickey and pulling my leg, she changed into a hostile argumentative person. Margaret often tried to escape from the house, searching for her mother. She didn't know who I was, but accused me of murdering her Mum.

I just about coped with all this, but the most difficult part of the package was cutting her toenails.

Finding a chiropodist was the first job I subcontracted, after insuring against the risk of a chiropodist with a broken jaw.

But my worst problem is loneliness. I miss terribly our lovely chatter together. It's ten years since I had any meaningful conversation with Margaret.

One nurse said I had 'carers syndrome' – a tendency to run to the gate and drag in the first passer-by, just for a quick chat.

How do I – and thousands of others – cope? Mainly by always keeping busy, so there's no time to feel sad. It's like a bereavement. The person I knew has gone, for ever. But after 56 years together I can't stop loving the new, incapable, incontinent, incoherent, immobile Margaret who sleeps for 22 hours every day. I make sure that she's clean and comfortable, warm and well fed. Margaret still enjoys her food – 'food comes first' was always her motto!

I've learned a lot from our carers, nurses and doctors. But sometimes, living at the coalface, I have to explain the effects and management of Alzheimer's to the health professionals.

So, how am I after 13 years of care? I grieve for some part of every day. But I feel fulfillment, because so far I have coped. I keep active. There's always something to do. Adrenalin keeps on churning round.

Finally, I wonder if government realises how much we unpaid family carers save the country? Without us, care homes and hospitals would overflow; the cost would bankrupt the NHS and the country. What might help? Sometimes we need a rest. We have to keep going, 24/7, day after day, week after week, year after year. This year (2011) I had a five day break, my first holiday in over 12 years. We see on TV how other people have holidays; but this is impossible for many family carers. One serious problem is paying for extra care in the home. A few years ago there was a government scheme called 'TAKE A BREAK' but the money wasn't ring-fenced. This scheme should be re-introduced, with proper safeguards to make sure that <u>family carers</u> actually benefit.

I've talked about separating the job from the emotions. But, Minister, I ask you and all the healthcare professionals here today, to direct both your jobs <u>and</u> your emotions towards caring for the vast army of family carers.

We depend on your support, Minister.

And please never forget, Sir,

– <u>YOU</u> depend on <u>US</u>!

Thank you, ladies and gentlemen.

Meet the Author

Front Line Alzheimer's

Meet the Author

"Caring is my fifth or even sixth profession," said Tom Wearden who has been a 24/7 carer since 1998 when his wife Margaret started on her Alzheimer's journey. Tom, a Chartered Engineer, with a degree in electrical engineering, has been an RNVR Officer, a development engineer, a sales engineer, a company manager, a business consultant and a freelance writer. "Perhaps there are more that I have forgotten. At least I am accustomed to new challenges!"

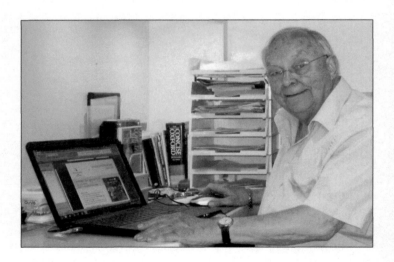

After many years in industry Tom became an independent consultant in 1980. "This gave me freedom to develop my interest in writing. I found a niche market producing company profiles and features for technical journals. In the next 17 years I wrote several hundred articles, many based on interviews with MDs - a lonely bunch who sometimes don't have anyone to talk to, so open up happily to an older writer who appreciates their problems."

Whilst caring for Margaret, Tom's creative, hands-on interests have provided welcome relief. He paints, plays jazzy piano improvisations on standards, and continues to write. "My latest project is collaboration with author Joy R Hartley on *Tales of Harina,* a series of five children's books." The first, *Harina: the Special Girl*, was published in February 2013.

"Ability to think like a child is vital when writing for young people, while understanding the unspoken needs of an advanced dementia sufferer means using common sense with compassion.

"When switching between my many roles I sometimes think of a book about method acting, read when I was both a mad scientist and a budding thespian, in my late teens: Stanislavski's *An Actor Prepares*. Perhaps this helped me prepare for all the changes throughout my fulfilling and varied life."

The joy of giving
with Harina books.

Children's books from Harina & Co. (Publications) Ltd.

Buy on line: www.harina-hanga.com
email: joy@harina-hanga.com

Follow on: www.twitter.com/harinahanga
www.facebook.com/harinahanga

Harina: the Special Girl

by Joy R. Hartley in collaboration with Tom Wearden

The first book in the *Tales of Harina* series.   ISBN 978-0-9575386-0-3

Harina®, a beautiful African girl whose favourite possession is a soft, comforting blanket, given by her grandmother when she was born, is befriended by a crested guinea fowl, who she calls **Hanga**®. These rare, wild birds are believed to bring good fortune. Together they have a magical adventure in which Harina® learns about *the joy of giving*.

Harina and the Doctor Bird

by Joy R Hartley in collaboration with Tom Wearden.

The second book in the *Tales of Harina* series

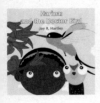

Harina® comes home from school to find Mummy poorly. She often thinks about her last adventure with the crested guinea fowl Hanga®, her favourite bird, where she saw the Doctor Bird and the Nurse Bird helping a poorly friend. 'Could they help Mummy? If only I could talk to them . . . .' she wondered. Then, as she drifted off into sleep, there was a tapping at the window . . . and Harina's® next adventure began.

PUBLISHED BY:

Harina & Co. (Publications) Ltd.
8, Allingham Court
26 Durham Avenue
Bromley, Kent, BR2 0QB

DISTRIBUTORS:

York Publishing Services Ltd.
64 Hallfield Road, Layerthorpe
York YO31 7ZQ
01904 431213